THE SUPER AGING WORKBOOK

DAVID CRAVIT
AND LARRY WOLF

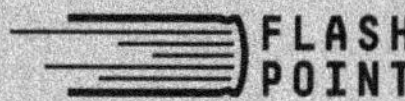

Published by Flashpoint™ Books, Seattle
www.flashpointbooks.com

Produced by Girl Friday Productions

Design: Paul Barrett and Rachel Marek
Development & editorial: Jessica Allen
Production editorial: Kylee Hayes
Project management: Emilie Sandoz-Voyer

ISBN (paperback): 978-1-964721-21-7

Disclaimer: This book is for informational purposes only and is not a substitute for professional medical advice. Always check with your qualified healthcare providers with any questions or concerns regarding a medical condition.

CONTENTS

DISCOVER THE 7 ESSENTIALS TO GETTING OLDER WITHOUT GETTING OLD

INTRODUCTION

Take a look at the following statements. Mark a *T* next to those that are true for you and an *F* next to those that are false.

T / F You plan to retire, or did retire, at age 65.

T / F You expect to live another 10–15 years following retirement.

T / F You anticipate experiencing worsening physical and mental health, sooner or later, so you're not planning to do much.

T / F You'll spend your days minimizing your suffering to achieve a relatively pain-free and dignified path to the finish line.

T / F You assume that you'll gradually start to slow down and withdraw from the world, declining offers to travel, socialize, or take up a new hobby.

T / F You accept ageism as a part of life.

T / F You think getting older beats the alternative, but otherwise doesn't have too many positives.

Which statements ring true to you? Some? All? None? These statements form the core of what we call **DefaultAging**.

Default aging still dominates healthcare, economics, housing, business, and virtually every aspect of how our society is organized. It sees "old" as a condition that kicks in, almost abruptly, when you reach the traditional retirement age of 65.

In truth, people are living longer. Someone turning 65 today can look forward to at least another 15 years, maybe a lot more. In 2024, the 85-plus population in the USA was close to 7 million people. The fastest-growing age group, in percentage terms, is centenarians!

But we think longevity can mean—should mean—much more than that. That's where **SuperAging** comes in. It's a totally new way to view what aging actually is: not just mathematically more years, but different years, with dramatically different characteristics. Instead of a relatively short, painful period of decline, aging now becomes a dynamic, positive time of life. Instead of mere survival, there are growth, development, new possibilities, and achievements.

Welcome to the SuperAging revolution, in which you get older without getting "old"!

NOBEL LAUREATE AT 97

Dr. John B. Goodenough made a groundbreaking contribution to the development of lithium-ion batteries, a technology that powers everything from smartphones to electric vehicles. While he had a long and distinguished career, his most notable achievement came when he was awarded the Nobel Prize in Chemistry in 2019 at the age of 97, making him the oldest Nobel laureate thus far.

HOW TO USE THIS BOOK

This workbook is full of actionable information and practical, simple exercises that will help you transform your relationship to yourself and to aging.

Many of you may have read our book *SuperAging*, so some of the concepts we discuss may be familiar to you. You can certainly work through this workbook while reading *SuperAging*, or you can use this workbook as a stand-alone resource. Our emphasis here is on taking easy, concrete steps toward becoming a SuperAger. Put another way: *SuperAging* explains the mindset, going deep into the research and science, while *The SuperAging Workbook* lays out the essential behaviors and helps you develop the habits you need to succeed.

You don't need to go to the gym or buy a bunch of fancy equipment. All you need is a pencil or pen, along with a willingness to put in the effort.

Each chapter deals with one of the different pillars of SuperAging and includes a mix of activities that will let you immediately apply the information you've learned to create a sustainable, lifelong SuperAging program of your own.

Begin with chapter 1, which outlines the seven *A*'s of SuperAging. Then turn to the "Attitude" and "Awareness" chapters, which provide a foundation for the chapters that follow. Having the right Attitude is crucial (chapter 2), as is developing a plan for learning more about the SuperAging topics that interest you (chapter 3). The remaining chapters can be done in whatever order makes sense to you.

While some activities are meant to be completed in one sitting, others will require ongoing effort. You may even wish to repeat some activities in the weeks and months to come. Feel free to use a notes app on your phone or keep a separate notebook for tracking your progress.

ACCOUNTABILITY IS THE 8TH A

SuperAgers don't simply absorb new information. They actively apply it to their lives. Spend a few minutes considering your goals for this workbook, and write them in the space below. If helpful, you could also jot down your plan for tackling this workbook, such as going through one chapter per week or month.

CHAPTER 1

THE 7 *A*'S OF SUPERAGING

THE SEVEN PILLARS OF SUPERAGING

We've identified seven critical pillars that, collectively, enable you to switch from the narrow DefaultAging mindset to the wider, infinitely more exciting SuperAging lens. We call them the seven *A*'s of SuperAging: Attitude, Awareness, Activity, Accomplishment, Autonomy, Attachment, and Avoidance (of certain negative factors).

1. **Attitude:** This is the underpinning of the entire SuperAging revolution. SuperAgers couple a positive attitude with a concrete vision of the future. They believe that they still have time to do a lot, and there's a lot they want to do.
2. **Awareness:** SuperAgers are active seekers and consumers of information. As importantly, they take an organized, systematic approach to information-gathering.

3. **Activity:** Staying active means exercising the body and the brain. SuperAgers like to learn new things and explore new approaches to nutrition, fitness, brain health, and overall wellness.
4. **Accomplishment:** SuperAgers have goals and plans to achieve them. They want to keep accomplishing things, whether in the workforce, by volunteering, by deepening their relationships, or in some other area.
5. **Autonomy:** SuperAgers value autonomy, ideally for the remainder of their lives. SuperAgers consider both physical autonomy, including aging in place, as well as financial autonomy.
6. **Attachment:** Loneliness and social isolation can seriously harm health and lifespan, so SuperAgers proactively cultivate existing relationships as well as seek additional opportunities for connection.
7. **Avoidance:** SuperAgers are aware of negative factors to avoid or combat, particularly ageism, fraud, and scams.

Embracing all seven pillars is your best path to SuperAging. But the first two—Attitude and Awareness—are necessary precursors for the remaining five. Each of those deal with a more specific issue (health and wellness, career and retirement, self-determination, social connectivity, and circumventing negative forces). But without the necessary Attitude or an efficient system for maintaining Awareness, you won't be able to fully explore the other issues and utilize the other tools.

All are interdependent. All are synergistic. Each is necessary and each reinforces the others, building a complete SuperAging program. With the seven *A*'s, you'll change from "manage the decline" to "accomplish so much more."

Here's how the elements are interrelated:

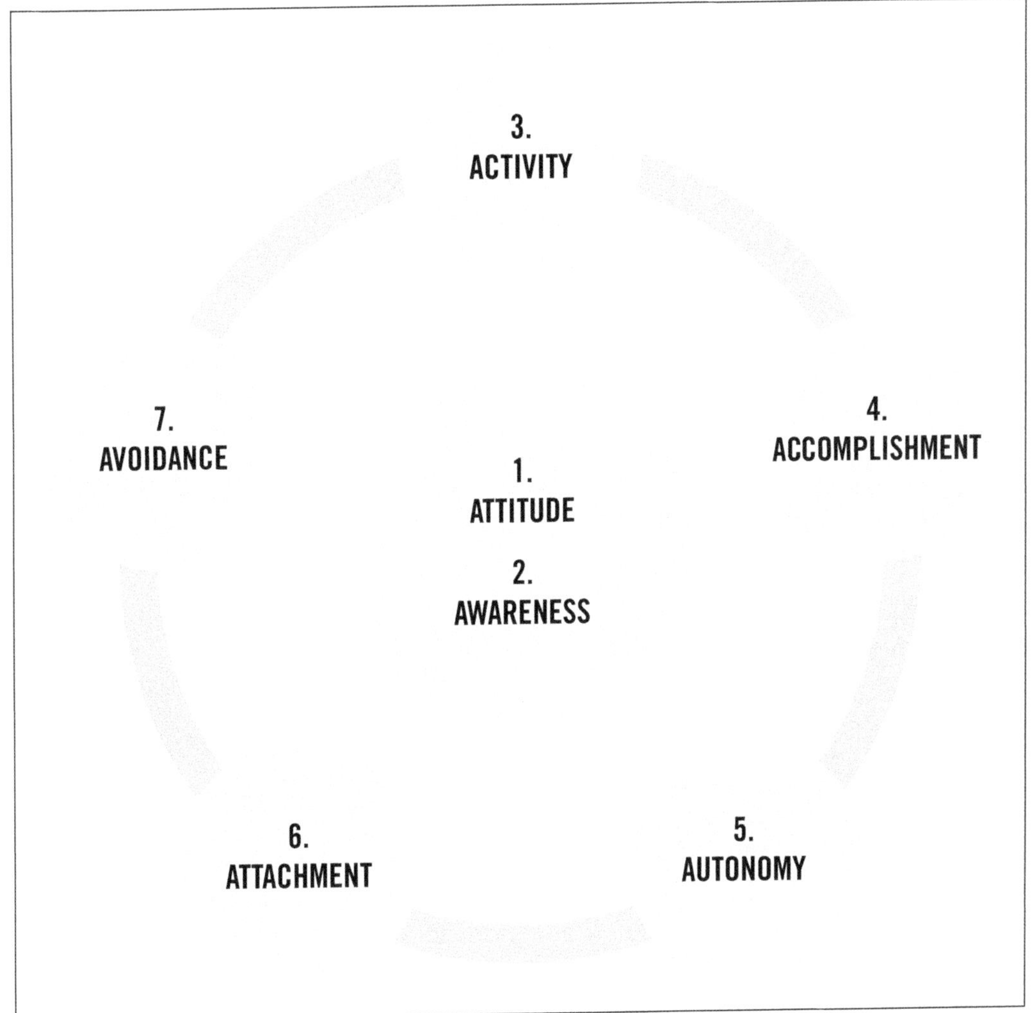

Shifting into a SuperAger requires consistent attention to *all* the *A*'s. By broadening your agenda, you set yourself up to maximize the potential of what could easily be 20 or 30 years (or more) of lifespan after the age of 65. This is how you "get older without getting old," how you live with purpose and energy and fulfillment.

You may be a DefaultAger now—not because you've done anything wrong but because it just kind of crept up on you, or it seems like that's the way things have to be. But you can be a SuperAger instead. Let's get started!

CHARACTERISTICS OF SUPERAGERS

What follows is a list of characteristics of SuperAgers. Circle those that apply to you at the present moment.

Positive

Active

Involved

Curious

Goal-oriented

Invested in your own health and care management

Willing to act as self-advocate

Confident

Enthusiastic about keeping fit, mentally and physically

Excited about the future

Eager for new experiences

Engaged with the world around you

Putting in effort to maintain or develop relationships

Interested in learning new things

Comfortable setting goals five, 10, and even 20 years into the future

Informed

Determined

Review the list again, paying attention to what you circled. What are the areas of strength for you? What are the areas of growth? Aim to get a baseline sense of your SuperAging Attitude.

Don't be discouraged if you didn't circle many characteristics at this point—after all, DefaultAging is a pervasive mindset, and you wouldn't have picked up this workbook if you weren't ready to transform.

As you move through the chapters, you might wish to revisit this list and notice how you're changing.

COMMUNITY HERO AT 72

Estella Pyfrom started picking beans alongside her parents at age 6. She eventually went to college and graduate school, then embarked on a 50-year career as an educator. Upon her retirement at age 72, she utilized her life savings to outfit a school bus as a mobile computer classroom. To date, Estella's Brilliant Bus has helped more than 500,000 kids and adults in under-resourced communities in South Florida develop computer literacy.

WHO ARE YOUR SUPERAGING ROLE MODELS?

Now that you're starting to see the distinctions between DefaultAging and SuperAging, consider the people in your life who exemplify SuperAging. They could be people you know well, such as family members or friends, or they could be celebrities or influencers. We've also included profiles of SuperAgers throughout this workbook for additional inspiration.

Use this space to write down your SuperAging role models. What makes them SuperAgers and worth emulating?

Pick one or two from your list. What is a habit or personality trait they have that you can incorporate into your own life today?

DON'T FORGET THE COMPANION WEBSITE, SUPERAGINGNEWS.COM!

If you've read *SuperAging*, then you know that one of our goals is to curate the vast amount of information on the topic of SuperAging. There is a constant stream of new discoveries in science, products, and resources; "the longevity business" is not only real but booming and growing, and SuperAgers need an easy resource for staying current and updated.

That's the role of our website, SuperAgingNews.com. Think of it as an essential companion to this workbook. It's where we will update the information provided in these chapters, plus bring you more in-depth coverage of the topics, including videos, podcasts, and even interactive surveys where you can express your own ideas and meet other like-minded SuperAgers. You'll also find a free e-newsletter that brings the freshest information and ideas directly into your email inbox.

Be sure to visit the website and bookmark it!

CHAPTER 2

ATTITUDE

WHAT ATTITUDE HAS TO DO WITH AGING

There is now strong, research-based evidence that a positive mental attitude contributes directly to a longer lifespan. In a study involving 70,000 people who were followed for 10 to 30 years, researchers at Boston University School of Medicine found that optimistic people can live up to 15% longer than pessimistic people.

The Baltimore Longitudinal Study of Aging (BLSA), initiated in 1958, is one of the longest-running studies on human aging. It has tracked the health data of around 1,500 volunteer subjects aged 17 to 49 over six decades, providing invaluable insights into the aging process. Findings from the BLSA show that people who maintain a positive outlook on aging tend to have better health outcomes. For instance, participants with optimistic attitudes about aging were found to have lower rates of cardiovascular disease, better cognitive function, and greater physical mobility. These findings help underscore the significant role of mindset in determining aging trajectories.

Or consider this study from the Yale School of Public Health, which started in 1975 with 1,000 subjects having an average age of 63. They were asked to agree or disagree with statements about aging. (For example, "As you get older, you are less useful.") They were then followed and their health outcomes were tracked for almost 30 years, until 2002. The average person with a positive attitude had almost a 50% higher remaining lifespan than the pessimists.

Having the right Attitude is fundamental to SuperAging.

MAKE ATTITUDE A PART OF YOUR SUPERAGING PROGRAM

In this section, you will learn how to:

- ❑ **Understand the foundation of SuperAging.** The world in which we're aging is different from the world of our parents, grandparents, and great-grandparents.
- ❑ **Gain a macro and micro outlook.** Develop a new perspective on your own tendencies and attitudes.
- ❑ **Be more optimistic.** Yes, optimism can be learned!
- ❑ **Reduce stress.** Too much stress can lead to excess cortisol, which, in turn, can cause inflammation that undermines overall health, affects mental well-being, and exacerbates chronic conditions.

UNDERSTAND THE FOUNDATION OF SUPERAGING

The foundation of the SuperAging Attitude has two elements.

1. **Longevity.** How long can we live? What is objectively realistic?

The reality of dramatically longer lifespans is destroying the DefaultAging model. Even if, for the sake of simplicity, we kept 65 as the jumping-off point for what comes after middle age, we're now looking at a very possible scenario of 25 SuperAging years, perhaps even more. So it makes no sense to treat those years as if they had nothing else to offer but warding off age-related pain and mitigating decline. Now you do have time to make new plans, set new goals, accomplish new things.

Longevity, then, is the primary driver of SuperAging because longevity has increasingly become the reality of what comes after middle age.

2. **Who is doing the aging?** What has our life experience been so far? What are our accumulated learnings, attitudes, and responses to other challenges and opportunities?

Different generations have different attitudes toward aging. We have to accept, up front, that generational comparisons can never be precisely accurate (or completely fair). Obviously, not every single Baby Boomer is exactly the same. That said, there is a wealth of behavioral research that identifies certain attitudes and behaviors that predominate within a particular generation compared to another generation, and that arise from the unique circumstances and life experiences of that generation. In the 21st century, there has been a cultural pushback against DefaultAging and stereotypes, largely led by the Baby Boomer generation. Whatever generation you belong to, your attitude about aging is informed by an array of factors.

WHAT'S YOUR GENERATION'S ATTITUDE TOWARD AGING?

Silent Generation, Baby Boomers, Generation X—each generation has its own attitudes about aging, which may or may not align with your attitude or with the SuperAging Attitude. Use this space to describe your generation's commonly accepted attitude toward aging. Do you hold a similar or different attitude from your generational peers? Why or why not?

HIP-HOP ARTIST AT 56

Upon releasing his 14th album in 2024, rapper and actor LL Cool J told the *Independent*, "Nothing lasts forever—but it can definitely last a lifetime." He began rapping at age 10 and scored his first hit record at age 16. After 40 years in hip-hop, though, the musician still has a lot to say and plans to keep saying it, citing curiosity and empathy as important factors in artistic innovation.

GET A SENSE OF YOUR ATTITUDE

Evaluate yourself with regard to the following statements, which relate to longevity and generational beliefs.

For each statement, choose ***5*** if you ***Strongly Agree***; choose ***4*** if you ***Somewhat Agree***; choose ***3*** if you're neutral (you ***Neither Agree nor Disagree***); choose ***2*** if you ***Somewhat Disagree***; choose ***1*** if you ***Strongly Disagree***.

I have time to make serious and satisfying plans.	5	4	3	2	1
I want to continue my professional development.	5	4	3	2	1
I want to keep working.	5	4	3	2	1
I want to keep on being influential.	5	4	3	2	1
If I stay on top of things, I can live a lot longer.	5	4	3	2	1

All the seven *A*'s of SuperAging are interconnected and mutually supportive. Nowhere is this truer than on the topic of Attitude. Whatever you brought with you before you started reading, be assured that a more positive outlook will be your rock-solid foundation in approaching all components of SuperAging.

REFLECT ON YOUR ATTITUDE

Look at your answers to the statements about Attitude. Did you vehemently agree—or disagree—with any of the statements? What surprised you about your overall attitude toward SuperAging?

Hard as it might be, try not to judge yourself. By virtue of working through the content of this workbook, you're already strengthening the foundation of a pro–SuperAging Attitude.

GAIN A MACRO OUTLOOK

Let's start with what you know or think about aging itself. Below are a series of statements. For each one, write down the number that comes closest to your current belief or feeling. Plan to repeat the quiz again after you've finished the book to see if your outlook has changed. You'll want to use another color of pen or pencil when you take the quiz for a second time.

For each statement, choose ***5*** if you ***Strongly Agree***; choose ***4*** if you ***Somewhat Agree***; choose **3** if you're neutral (you ***Neither Agree nor Disagree***); choose **2** if you ***Somewhat Disagree***; choose ***1*** if you ***Strongly Disagree***.

People may be living longer, but we've probably pushed longevity as far as it can go.	5	4	3	2	1
I don't believe I should have to retire at 65; there's lots more I can accomplish.	5	4	3	2	1
I rely on my doctor to keep me informed of the latest in medical and diet information.	5	4	3	2	1
I already have set clear goals and objectives for 10 years out.	5	4	3	2	1
I check the nutritional content of all the food I eat.	5	4	3	2	1
I consider myself an optimist.	5	4	3	2	1
I have a good understanding of how exercise can benefit my health and lifespan.	5	4	3	2	1
Despite all the hype about longevity, I think most people are still aging the way they always did.	5	4	3	2	1
I like to pick unfamiliar destinations for my holiday travel.	5	4	3	2	1
I don't see the point of having a bucket list. For me, at least, there probably won't be enough time.	5	4	3	2	1
My faith matters to me.	5	4	3	2	1
I'd like to start a business of my own someday.	5	4	3	2	1
I am very worried about winding up in a nursing home.	5	4	3	2	1
Even if I could live beyond 100, I don't think I'd want to.	5	4	3	2	1

I am very interested in alternative and holistic medicine.	5	4	3	2	1
I enjoy technology and try to keep up with the latest developments.	5	4	3	2	1
I have already set clear goals and objectives for 20 years out.	5	4	3	2	1
I've had a long and happy life, and it's time to relax and do nothing.	5	4	3	2	1
I don't think there's much I can do to change my life.	5	4	3	2	1
There are many new things I'd still like to learn.	5	4	3	2	1
I don't see any reason I shouldn't expect to be at my grandchildren's weddings.	5	4	3	2	1
There's a lot of buzz about "reversing aging," but I don't think it will ever really happen.	5	4	3	2	1
I regularly seek out news about science and tech discoveries.	5	4	3	2	1
I have already set clear goals and objectives for 30 years out.	5	4	3	2	1
I am concerned about ageism and the tendency to discount what older generations can still contribute to society.	5	4	3	2	1

As you can see, the quiz offers a mix of positive and negative statements: some describe a high state of awareness and concern, while others, a low state; some describe an active and optimistic view of the future, while others, a more passive or even defeatist one.

The benefit of the exercise is that it gets you to think about these topics all at once, and to reflect on their role in the aging process. These may be questions you haven't thought seriously about, or at all. What we're trying to do here, very simply, is to help you tune in to the idea of aging as a whole and begin to place it in the context of your own knowledge, attitudes, and beliefs.

There are no right or wrong answers and no need to add up or average your scores. The *thought process itself* is the whole point.

REFLECT ON YOUR MACRO OUTLOOK

What do you already know about these topics, how strongly do you feel about them, and do they trigger any other thoughts or ideas about aging? Taking the quiz before you've read anything further will bring the DefaultAging versus SuperAging landscape into sharper focus and cause you to consider, and become more sensitive to, some of the key issues and options as they might affect you. That's what we're trying to accomplish at this stage.

Take this opportunity to reflect on your macro outlook. In what ways does it reflect a SuperAging Attitude? Where do you have room for improvement?

GAIN A MICRO OUTLOOK

Before you take the next quiz, ask yourself if you are more of an optimist or a pessimist. What do you think, and why? What life experiences and choices make you answer the way you did?

In this section, we look at the optimistic and pessimistic factors that *you* bring to the party based on your individual personality—independent of the topic of aging. We present the Life Orientation Test, originally developed at Carnegie Mellon University in 1985 and widely used for professional psychological assessments.

For each statement, choose **5** if you ***Strongly Agree***; choose **4** if you ***Somewhat Agree***; choose **3** if you're neutral (you ***Neither Agree nor Disagree***); choose **2** if you ***Somewhat Disagree***; choose ***1*** if you ***Strongly Disagree.***

I can find something meaningful or significant in everyday events.	5	4	3	2	1
There is a reason for everything that happens to me.	5	4	3	2	1
There is no ultimate meaning or purpose in life.	5	4	3	2	1
There is no point in searching for meaning in life.	5	4	3	2	1
No matter how painful the situation is, life is still worth living.	5	4	3	2	1
The meaning of life is to "eat, drink, and be happy."	5	4	3	2	1
What really matters to me is to pursue a higher purpose or calling, regardless of personal cost.	5	4	3	2	1
I would rather be a happy pig than a sad saint.	5	4	3	2	1
I am willing to sacrifice personal interests for the greater good.	5	4	3	2	1
Personal happiness and success are more important to me than achieving inner goodness and moral excellence.	5	4	3	2	1

YOUR TOTAL SCORE: ______________
YOUR AVERAGE (total / 10): ______________

- If your score averaged **less than 3**, you are more of a **pessimist**.
- If you scored **between 3 and 4**, you're **neutral** and could go either way, depending on the situation.
- If you scored **4 or more**, you're inclined toward **optimism**.

REFLECT ON YOUR MICRO OUTLOOK

Flip back to p. 17, where you noted whether you considered yourself an optimist or pessimist. Compare your answer there to your score here. Maybe you didn't need a test to tell you that you are more of a pessimist than an optimist. Or maybe you weren't sure, and you find your score to be revealing. Were you surprised by your results? Why or why not?

LEARN TO BE AN OPTIMIST

The presence of optimism or pessimism, whatever any genetic predisposition, is still heavily dependent on experience and learning. You experience situations, you form judgments (positive or negative) about likely outcomes, events prove you right or wrong, and you adapt your attitudes accordingly. These accumulate into an attitudinal underpinning that tilts toward optimism or pessimism.

But that underpinning is constantly being applied to new situations and new circumstances. The process is dynamic, not static. In short, optimism can be learned. Thanks to the work of psychologist, educator, and author Dr. Martin Seligman, who pioneered an approach to dealing with adversity that is still taught today, the field of positive psychology has exploded. There are literally hundreds of "positivity" apps available in both the Google and Apple stores. We urge you to check them out and try some for yourself.

You can also use the checklist below as a guide for developing a more optimistic outlook. Check or circle the areas you might need to concentrate on improving, or come back to this page as you try each strategy to mark your progress.

- ❑ **Be kind to yourself.**
- ❑ **Reduce stress.**
- ❑ **Do activities you enjoy.**
- ❑ **Anticipate positive events.**
- ❑ **Surround yourself with positive people.**
- ❑ **Reframe negative thoughts.**
- ❑ **Avoid catastrophizing (focusing on the worst possible outcome).**

Which strategy seems most doable for you? Remember that you don't have to employ every strategy at once. Instead, pick a strategy and try it for a week or month.

PRACTICE AN ATTITUDE OF GRATITUDE

Cultivate an attitude of gratitude by focusing on the positive and expressing appreciation for the blessings you have. Experts say the ability to shrug off life's small frustrations can go a long way toward less stress and improved overall mental well-being—which can contribute to a stronger immune function and better cardiovascular health.

Make a list of everything you're grateful for today, big or small. Continue to add to this list as you develop and practice your gratitude attitude.

CONSIDER WHAT'S GOTTEN BETTER

What's getting better as you get older? We love this question, because it helps you reframe the inevitability of change. Consider what's changed for the better for you as you've gotten older. Be as specific as possible. Once you've considered your own life, you could even widen your lens and journal about what's gotten better about the world as you've aged.

REDUCE STRESS

While it's next to impossible to eliminate stress entirely, there are key strategies to manage it and mitigate its impact on our health and well-being.

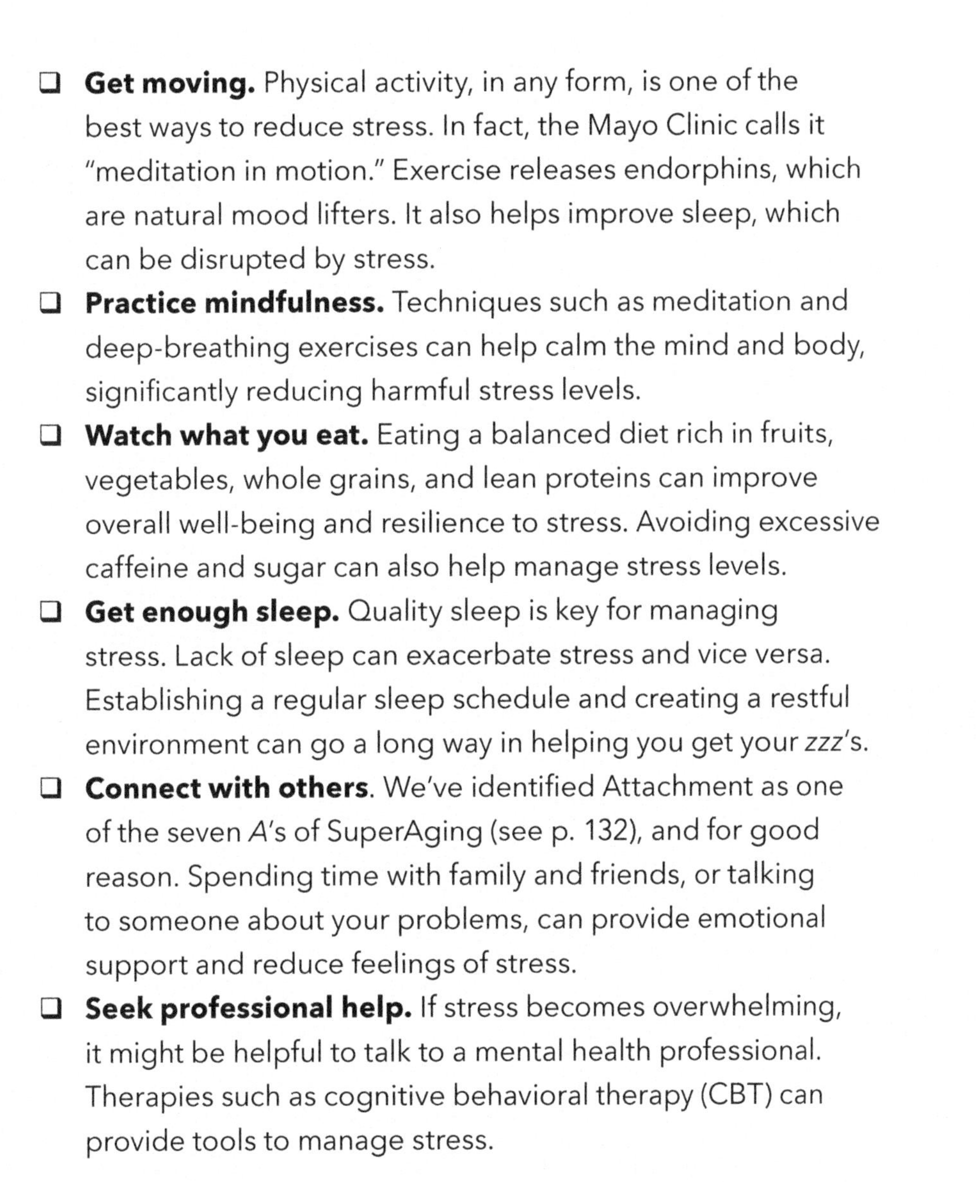

- ☐ **Get moving.** Physical activity, in any form, is one of the best ways to reduce stress. In fact, the Mayo Clinic calls it "meditation in motion." Exercise releases endorphins, which are natural mood lifters. It also helps improve sleep, which can be disrupted by stress.
- ☐ **Practice mindfulness.** Techniques such as meditation and deep-breathing exercises can help calm the mind and body, significantly reducing harmful stress levels.
- ☐ **Watch what you eat.** Eating a balanced diet rich in fruits, vegetables, whole grains, and lean proteins can improve overall well-being and resilience to stress. Avoiding excessive caffeine and sugar can also help manage stress levels.
- ☐ **Get enough sleep.** Quality sleep is key for managing stress. Lack of sleep can exacerbate stress and vice versa. Establishing a regular sleep schedule and creating a restful environment can go a long way in helping you get your *zzz*'s.
- ☐ **Connect with others**. We've identified Attachment as one of the seven *A*'s of SuperAging (see p. 132), and for good reason. Spending time with family and friends, or talking to someone about your problems, can provide emotional support and reduce feelings of stress.
- ☐ **Seek professional help.** If stress becomes overwhelming, it might be helpful to talk to a mental health professional. Therapies such as cognitive behavioral therapy (CBT) can provide tools to manage stress.

Chronic stress is a serious health issue that can affect almost every aspect of our lives—as well as our long-term longevity. As you'll see in coming chapters, many of these stress-reduction strategies appear again as part of our SuperAging program.

STRESS LESS

Write down everything that's causing you stress right now, then carefully review the list. The goal isn't to eliminate every stressor, which would be impossible. Instead, circle those that are in your control.

TAKE ACTION

Review whatever you've circled. List concrete actions you can take to reduce or eliminate those stressors. Remember, too, that you have more control than you might otherwise think. For example, if you're dismayed by a political situation, you can volunteer for a campaign.

NOTICE WHAT'S GOOD

Spend a few minutes at the end of each day recalling at least one Good Thing that happened. A Good Thing can be as simple as watching a bird take flight, catching a green light, or getting a wave from a young child—and, in fact, simple is better, so you can start to see how many seemingly ordinary moments in our lives are actually quite joyful. The goal is to train yourself to find and appreciate the joy in the everyday.

Date:

Good Thing:

Date:

Good Thing:

Date:

Good Thing:

Date:

Good Thing:

Date:

Good Thing:

Date:

Good Thing:

Date:

Good Thing:

HARNESS THE POWER OF ANTICIPATION

Studies in 2015 and 2017 found that anticipating positive events has big benefits for our mental health and well-being at the neurological level. The data is clear: Getting excited about something helps foster a positive attitude. What are you looking forward to? Use this space to jot down a few things you're excited about. Ideally you'll want to have a mix of time horizons, from next week to next month to next year to a few years from now.

ACTIVITY/EVENT	TIME FRAME

REFRAME NEGATIVE THOUGHTS

Tap into the brain's plasticity and ability to change by teaching yourself to reframe negative thoughts. We all have them, of course, whether worries about our families, broader concerns about society or the planet, or regrets about a past experience. Too often, though, a negative thought starts to spin out. Like a tornado, it picks up everything in its path. Learning to reframe negative thoughts can stop this negativity spiral and help you gain perspective. First, challenge your negative thought—what is your evidence for thinking that? Could there be other explanations? Then, replace your negative thought with a positive thought. For example, say your negative thought is: "Technology today is too complicated and I'll never figure it out." You could think about all the new technologies you *have* learned to use and reframe that as: "Technology has changed a lot in my life and I've changed with it, learning so many new things."

Jot down your own negative thoughts, then reframe them.

Negative thought:

Reframe:

Negative thought:

Reframe:

Negative thought:

Reframe:

KEY TAKEAWAYS

Use this space to write down your key takeaways, notes to self, and anything else you'd like to remember from this chapter.

NEXT STEPS

Remember the honorary eighth pillar: *Accountability.* Fill in the blanks, giving yourself a reasonable timeline. Be as specific as possible about the action and your reason(s) for undertaking it. Concrete whys help ensure follow-through.

In the next ____________________, I will ____.

I'm going to do this because ____.

I'm also excited to ____.

SCHEDULE YOUR HAPPINESS

The Greater Good Science Center, at the University of California, Berkeley, studies the science behind happiness, compassion, and other elements of a meaningful life. Every month the center produces a downloadable online calendar, with tips to try and links to related articles.

FIND IT HERE:
https://greatergood.berkeley.edu/topic/happiness

CHAPTER 3

AWARENESS

HOW TO STAY AWARE WHILE YOU AGE

Attitude and Awareness are the foundational necessities—the two bedrock *A*'s of SuperAging—because they equip us to engage with the other pillars, all of which are more specific in their roles and applications.

To fully maximize the promise of SuperAging, you need to start paying attention to how you are going to spend your next years. And that, in turn, means dealing with everything from retirement and personal reinvention to housing, financial strategies, relationships, technology . . . and more.

DefaultAgers are essentially passive about information. Their approach is mostly to let the information come to them as opposed to actively seeking it out. SuperAgers, in contrast, approach Awareness from a proactive point of view.

As a result of this attitude toward Awareness, SuperAgers are:

- ❑ **Reluctant to see "experts" as the sole source.** Instead, they seek other points of view. This might include other physicians, reputable medical websites, and even those who might have the same medical condition.
- ❑ **Determined to know and control their own personal health data.** SuperAgers are much more ready and willing to monitor and track key health metrics. For the SuperAger, Awareness extends to intimately knowing what is happening in their own body.
- ❑ **Ready to use multiple resources to get the information they need.** SuperAgers don't want to wait for the necessary information to come to them; they eagerly seek it out through every means available, particularly the internet.

CONSIDER YOUR AWARENESS ATTITUDE

When it comes to Awareness, do these statements currently apply to you? Why or why not? Be honest about your present point of view—and remember that DefaultAging attitudes are both pervasive and prevalent, so give yourself a break if you don't see yourself in these statements—yet.

Being informed is essential to SuperAging. Yet, if we start out by confronting the total information landscape—without doing any selecting, categorizing, or other organizing—it can look like a completely chaotic and intimidating jungle of topics. We need to make sure we're keeping an eye on topics of relevance to us. The best way to do that is to have an organized tracking system.

MAKE AWARENESS PART OF YOUR SUPERAGING PROGRAM

In this section, you will learn how to:

- ❑ **Create a list of SuperAging topics.**
- ❑ **Choose your sources.**
- ❑ **Select and store your content.**
- ❑ **Vet your sources.**

CREATE A LIST OF SUPERAGING TOPICS

The first step is to list the major SuperAging topics you'll be following. Of course, there are literally thousands of possibilities, but we recommend keeping it simple and using large and intuitive categories.

Those listed below play into at least one of the seven *A*'s; some touch on several. Circle or highlight those of interest to you.

1. **Diet:** Healthy eating, foods that promote longevity, recipes, and menu plans
2. **Fitness:** Physical and mental health, including exercise programs and brain-fitness programs
3. **Finance:** Investment strategies, financial independence
4. **Health:** Prevention and wellness, anti-aging research, new therapies, new products and services for monitoring and tracking
5. **Housing:** Aging in place and associated products and services, healthy locations for retirement, new concepts in retirement living and senior housing
6. **People:** Inspiring stories about SuperAgers, role models
7. **Relationships:** Social connectivity, apps, and other digital tools, creating new and existing networks
8. **Retirement:** Retirement planning, new forms of retirement (part-time, hybrid, second careers, and reinvention), new forms of ongoing activity (volunteering, mentoring), techniques for long-term planning
9. **Science:** Biomedical research, new projects, and discoveries related to slowing down, preventing, or reversing aging
10. **Social issues:** Politics, combating ageism, economic and demographic trends that influence the other topics
11. **Technology:** Age-tech (including telehealth and interactive monitoring), AI, robotics, cloud-based interconnected systems

Write down your list on the next page. Feel free to tweak, relabel, or redefine some of the categories to make them more descriptive or applicable to your particular priorities. You may also add, subtract, or regroup; as time goes on, it's inevitable that new topics will emerge.

CHOOSE YOUR SOURCES

Our list of topics gives us a consistent structure to organize the information landscape, but we also need a way to categorize all the sources from which information can flow. We quickly see that there are two types of sources:

1. **Core sources** that focus specifically on aging and related issues. These may be books, publications, websites, YouTube channels, blogs, podcasts, e-newsletters, or websites of aging-related organizations (e.g., AARP or, in Canada, CARP). Together, they represent a "core" list of sources that we will want to check on a regular basis.
2. **Intermittent sources** that do not focus exclusively on aging, but which may offer valuable information from time to time. The topic of aging is becoming so important that virtually all media—from *The New York Times* to *Newsweek* to *The Economist* to *Forbes*—regularly produce articles, blog posts, or videos with new and important information on one of our key topics.

CATEGORIZE YOUR SOURCES

Make a list of your current sources of information. Indicate whether the source is "core" or "intermittent."

When you finish working through the other exercises in this chapter, you can refer back to this list and see whether you need to add any sources to diversify your information streams.

SOURCE	CORE OR INTERMITTENT?		NOTES

SOURCE	CORE OR INTERMITTENT?		NOTES
	CORE	INT	
	CORE	INT	
	CORE	INT	
	CORE	INT	
	CORE	INT	
	CORE	INT	
	CORE	INT	
	CORE	INT	
	CORE	INT	
	CORE	INT	
	CORE	INT	
	CORE	INT	
	CORE	INT	
	CORE	INT	
	CORE	INT	
	CORE	INT	
	CORE	INT	
	CORE	INT	

SOURCE	CORE OR INTERMITTENT?		NOTES

ORGANIZE YOUR SOURCES AND TOPICS

Fill in the chart that follows, using your SuperAging topic and source lists. As your knowledge and interests expand, you might find that you want to

TOPICS	DESCRIPTION	"CORE GROUP" SOURCES	
		Books	Newspapers/ magazines
SUPERAGING	The whole topic overall		
DIET	Healthier eating; cooking; menu plans		
FITNESS	Exercise programs; best practices		
FINANCE	Investment; financial independence		
HEALTH	Prevention; treatment; overall wellness		
HOUSING	Aging in place		
PEOPLE	Human-interest stories; role models		

add sources to your core group. We included our SuperAging topics as well, given their importance to SuperAging overall.

"CORE GROUP" SOURCES			
Websites/ e-newsletters	Videos/podcasts	Apps	Other

TOPICS	DESCRIPTION	"CORE GROUP" SOURCES	
		Books	Newspapers/ magazines
RELATIONSHIPS	Social connectivity		
RETIREMENT	Retirement planning; second acts; career reinvention		
SCIENCE	Research into slowing down, preventing, and reversing aging		
SOCIAL ISSUES	Politics; economics; demographic trends		
TECHNOLOGY	AI, robots, age-tech		

"CORE GROUP" SOURCES			
Websites/ e-newsletters	Videos/podcasts	Apps	Other

SET UP YOUR INTERMITTENT SOURCES

Your core group of regularly scanned sources, hefty as it may be, represents only a fraction of the information that's out there on any given topic. There will be a virtual fire hose of articles, blogs, videos, podcasts, and so on coming from sources that are not listed in your core resources library. How do you keep track?

As mentioned, we generally keep an eye out for topics of interest to us—reading an article about age-tech when it appears in our local newspaper, for example. But we don't just wait for information to come to us. We also have a series of Google Alerts set up for important terms, including:

- ❑ BABY BOOMERS
- ❑ LIVING TO 100
- ❑ RETIREMENT
- ❑ WORKING PAST RETIREMENT
- ❑ AGE-TECH
- ❑ REVERSE AGING
- ❑ LONGEVITY
- ❑ REINVENTING AGING
- ❑ CENTENARIANS
- ❑ OUTLIVING YOUR MONEY
- ❑ HEALTH TECH
- ❑ AGEISM

The list may not look that big, and that's by design. You should keep the list small, especially at the beginning; you don't want to get overwhelmed by seeing hundreds of results piling up in your email inbox and be unable to deal with them. As you go along, you can drop certain search terms or add others, such as subtopics of subjects producing results that you find especially interesting or helpful.

MAKE A LIST OF YOUR SEARCH TERMS

Whenever something appears on the internet that matches one of your search terms, the service sends you an email alert and a link to where the term appears (article, video, podcast, etc.). You can specify how often you want to receive alerts. You can also let them accumulate in your email inbox and check them when convenient. The important thing is that the services are constantly examining the internet for new material that contains your search terms.

SELECT AND STORE YOUR CONTENT

Once you have your content pouring in, you need some method of selecting what to keep to review at your convenience. We recommend three digital note-taking tools for your consideration: Evernote, FuseBase (formerly known as Nimbus Note), and Notion. All three create a workspace where your selected content can be stored. Very importantly, since so much of that content will be in the form of a web page (be it an article, blog, podcast, or video), all three offer a browser plug-in that works as a "web clipper," enabling you to immediately save that web page directly into the workspace. No need to manually copy the material.

Do some research into productivity software and note-taking apps. Some are free, some have a fee, and some might work better in different browsers. List the results of your research or any follow-ups here.

CAPTURE SURPRISING FACTS

Use this space to capture the fun and surprising facts you're learning about SuperAging topics of interest to you. Refer to this list for reminders about further research, activities you wish to try, or behavior modifications you'd like to make.

VET YOUR SOURCES

No matter how we organize the inbound torrent or how cleverly we categorize and select and then store our selections in an orderly vault for later review and evaluation, the fact remains that some of it will be more reliable and some less reliable. That's just a fact of life in the internet age.

We recommend a very short and simple list of vetting practices:

- ❑ **Use social media only as a jumping-off point.** Social media should never be a source by itself. Social media can refer you to a source, which can then be viewed and evaluated.
- ❑ **Look at who is giving an endorsement.** If reviewers or endorsers have relevant credentials, it's more likely the content is reliable. Don't forget that "relevant credentials" may include being a fellow SuperAger. Is the endorser being paid for their endorsement? That's something to keep in mind.
- ❑ **Be wary of definitive conclusions around emerging data.** Be cautious of conclusions that are too definitive too early on, particularly when it comes to constantly updating science and research.
- ❑ **Trust reputable, proven sources.** Prefer sources that are backed by solid and documented research from blue-chip institutions. Be suspicious of "gurus" with oversimplified advice based solely on their own anecdotal experience.
- ❑ **Make room for differing opinions.** Don't be afraid of uncertainty, gray areas, or even contradictory evidence or conclusions. What you should be trying to do is weed out what is clearly bogus. There's plenty of room for differing opinions or emerging research that adds new light to subjects.
- ❑ **Make a habit of checking in with SuperAgingNews.com.** We've worked hard to patrol and analyze the jungle of information and curate the material that is most trustworthy and reliable on our companion website.

SOCIAL MEDIA AND SUPERAGING

For most people, social media plays a huge role in their daily lives. What social media sites do you check regularly? In what ways do—or can—your favorite social media sites support your SuperAging program?

JOIN US ON FACEBOOK

Join our SuperAging Community on Facebook to connect with like-minded SuperAgers and make your voice heard.

DEVELOP YOUR CHECKING CADENCE

At this point, you might be feeling overwhelmed, as if staying abreast of the latest developments is going to be a full-time job. It's important to remember that we're talking about Awareness here, not encyclopedic knowledge.

The simple act of periodically looking at your Awareness lists and charts from this chapter—even once every three or four weeks—provides an immediate reminder. In time, you'll start to develop a feel for how long it's been since you saw something or read something on a given topic, and whether you're generally up to date with the latest wisdom.

Your own interests and predispositions are important too. You'll soon find it's impossible to be equally aware of every topic, and that your level of attention will vary widely. There's nothing wrong with this! Remember, what you're comparing this to is a previous condition in which you had no list of topics, no list of sources, no systematic way of going after the information you need. By keeping it simple, you're more likely to get into the habit of checking up on a regular basis instead of being burdened by a task list that never quite gets satisfied. Being a SuperAger does require work, but it shouldn't be overly complex or burdensome.

Pick a few sources and topics from the previous pages, then fill in the chart below, including how often you'll check.

SOURCE	TOPIC	FREQUENCY
SuperAging News website	*SuperAging*	*Several times a week*
SuperAging News newsletter	*SuperAging*	*In my inbox, multiple times a week*

SOURCE	TOPIC	FREQUENCY

TRACK YOUR RECOMMENDATIONS

Keep track of book recommendations, websites you want to visit, podcasts you want to listen to, and other new content you want to explore here. Bookmark or put a sticky note on this page so you'll have it handy when you're shopping or browsing the internet.

BOOKS	NEWSPAPERS/MAGAZINES
WEBSITES/NEWSLETTERS	**VIDEOS/PODCASTS**
APPS	**OTHER**

KEY TAKEAWAYS

Use this space to write down your key takeaways, notes to self, and anything else you'd like to remember from this chapter.

NEXT STEPS

Remember the honorary eighth pillar: *Accountability.* Fill in the blanks, giving yourself a reasonable time horizon. Be as specific as possible about the action and your reason(s) for undertaking it. Concrete whys help ensure follow-through.

In the next ______________, I will ____
____.

I'm going to do this because ____
____.

I'm also excited to ____
____.

COLLEGE GRADUATE AT 102

Sarah Simpkins dropped out of Allen University, where she was studying to become a teacher, after getting pregnant with her first child in 1942. More than 80 years later, the 102-year-old earned a degree from Brightpoint Community College's Early Childhood Education program. To make the occasion even more significant, Simpkins graduated alongside her granddaughter.

CHAPTER 4

ACTIVITY

THE ACTIVITIES THAT MAKE YOU A SUPERAGER

Technically, everything you do could be called Activity, whether it deals with your body or your finances or your social network or your career. But in the context of SuperAging, we define Activity as meaning "physical or mental activity to promote health and well-being." This covers:

- Wellness (which encompasses overall health and disease prevention or mitigation)
- Diet and nutrition
- Exercise and physical fitness
- Brain health, especially prevention or mitigation of dementia / Alzheimer's disease

In choosing how best to navigate the forest of fact and judgment around Activity, we are guided by a few basic principles. Everything we present

- is endorsed by credible experts and, where possible, backed up by scientific research.
- can achieve positive results.
- is workable. You can do this!
- can be done at home. You can be a SuperAger without following complex systems or incurring high costs.
- is intended to serve as a road map, an aid, and hopefully, an inspiration toward learning more and keeping your knowledge up to date. But it's not a rigid system or set of rules requiring you to do every single thing. Most importantly, it is not intended to replace medical advice, so be sure to check with your doctor before following any particular diet or exercise program.

CONQUEROR OF MOUNT EVEREST AT 80

Born in 1932, Japanese alpinist Yūichirō Miura climbed Mount Everest three times, with his final summit in 2013 at the age of 80, making him the oldest person to reach the peak. He summited with his son by his side. Miura loved winter sports from a young age. Other alpine accomplishments include skiing down the tallest peaks of each of the seven continents by age 53.

MAKE ACTIVITY PART OF YOUR SUPERAGING PROGRAM

In this section, you will learn how to:

- ❑ **Recognize that the world has changed.** You have a lot more room to take action, and there are a lot more resources to help you.
- ❑ **Realize you have choices.** When it comes to health and wellness, start thinking like a consumer.
- ❑ **Join the broader conversation.** We're not suggesting you ignore your doctor's advice and abruptly follow the counsel of some fellow-sufferer patient on a website. But you should at least be familiar with the kind of dialogue that is going on there, the types of issues and ideas that are being put forward.
- ❑ **Be more proactive with your primary caregiver.** Do research ahead of your appointment and come armed with questions. Make notes and review them when you get home. Get copies of test results. Follow up as necessary.
- ❑ **Check if your health insurance provider includes P4P (pay for performance).** Also known as value-based payment, P4P creates models that attach both incentives and disincentives to provider performance, tying reimbursement to measurable results.
- ❑ **Keep up to date with new developments.** Use your Awareness trackers from chapter 3 to stay informed.

ENTER THE CHAT

Don't wait to join the broader conversation around a health condition you're managing or concerned about. Type "[condition] chat room" into your search bar. Scroll through your results, and find one or two that seem reputable. You might have to register to gain access. But once you're on the site, you can see fairly quickly whether it's a place in which you'd like to spend some time. If so, great. If not, go back to your search results and keep looking. You might also consider searching for Facebook groups that can help you connect to others in a similar situation as yours.

Use this space to make notes about favorite chat rooms, search results, groups, or screen names—just don't write down your passwords. If you're concerned about misinformation, see our guidance around vetting sources on p. 48.

WELLNESS TO-DOS

When it comes to wellness, what are your biggest areas of opportunity? Is it improving interactions with your doctor, switching your insurance, or something else? Write down your thoughts and wellness goals as a series of action items. We've also included a self-care cheat sheet to help guide your wellness goals.

SELF-CARE CHEAT SHEET

- ❑ **Stay physically active.**
- ❑ **Maintain social connections.**
- ❑ **Prioritize sleep.**
- ❑ **Practice mindfulness and relaxation techniques.**
- ❑ **Eat right.**
- ❑ **Find hobbies you love.**
- ❑ **Practice gratitude and positive thinking.**
- ❑ **Embrace self-care rituals.**
- ❑ **Seek professional support when needed.**

MAKE DIET AND NUTRITION PART OF YOUR SUPERAGING PROGRAM

- ☐ **Drink plenty of water.** Dehydration inhibits longevity, and causes more fatigue, a reduction in mental energy, and less efficient digestion. Aim for eight 8-ounce glasses of water per day, but check with your doctor.
- ☐ **Practice portion control.** A good way to eat in moderation is to control portion sizes.
- ☐ **Eat the "rainbow."** Vary what's on your plate, and try to consume as many brightly colored fruits and vegetables as possible. The Mediterranean diet, which emphasizes fruits, vegetables, and seafood, and de-emphasizes meat, is a good reference.
- ☐ **Consider the benefits of fasting.** Intermittent fasting has been shown to promote healthy aging. There are several recognized variations, including time-restricted fasting, when you only eat during a certain window (for example, 10:00 a.m.–6:00 p.m.).

DETERMINE YOUR PROTEIN NEEDS

Protein not only helps you feel full and reduces cravings, but it also helps you build and maintain muscle mass, lower your blood pressure, and prevent sarcopenia (muscle loss). While experts generally recommend that adults get 0.36 grams of protein per pound of body weight, some researchers have started suggesting that adults over the age of 65 should opt for even more protein: at least 0.45 to 0.54 grams per pound. Are you getting enough?

Take a look inside your cabinets and refrigerator and write down the amount of protein per serving in your favorite foods. Depending on what you discover, consider tweaking serving sizes or incorporating new foods into your diet.

FOOD	PROTEIN PER SERVING

PRACTICE PORTION CONTROL

A good way to eat in moderation is to control portion sizes. People usually eat everything they dish out, so if you have smaller portions, you'll automatically be reducing the tendency to overeat. Here are few suggestions for how to limit portion size, along with space for you to write down how the strategy worked for you. We've included extra space, since you might have to try these strategies at different meals or with different foods to figure out what's best for you.

Use a smaller plate.

Meal/food:
Result:
How full were you on a scale of 1 (still hungry) to 5 (stuffed)?

Meal/food:
Result:
How full were you on a scale of 1 (still hungry) to 5 (stuffed)?

Meal/food:
Result:
How full were you on a scale of 1 (still hungry) to 5 (stuffed)?

Adhere to the serving size listed on the package.

Meal/food:
Result:
How full were you on a scale of 1 (still hungry) to 5 (stuffed)?

Meal/food:
Result:
How full were you on a scale of 1 (still hungry) to 5 (stuffed)?

Meal/food:
Result:
How full were you on a scale of 1 (still hungry) to 5 (stuffed)?

Divide your plate as follows: half for vegetables or salad, a quarter for protein (meat, fish, poultry, eggs), and a quarter for carbs (whole grains, starchy vegetables).

Meal/food:
Result:
How full were you on a scale of 1 (still hungry) to 5 (stuffed)?

Meal/food:
Result:
How full were you on a scale of 1 (still hungry) to 5 (stuffed)?

Meal/food:
Result:
How full were you on a scale of 1 (still hungry) to 5 (stuffed)?

Eat more slowly. It can take at least 15 minutes to realize you're full.

Meal/food:
Result:
How full were you on a scale of 1 (still hungry) to 5 (stuffed)?

Meal/food:
Result:
How full were you on a scale of 1 (still hungry) to 5 (stuffed)?

Meal/food:
Result:
How full were you on a scale of 1 (still hungry) to 5 (stuffed)?

A Harvard study showed that women who had two or more servings of berries a week delayed memory decline by as much as two and a half years and decreased their risk of a heart attack.

STOCK YOUR SUPERAGING KITCHEN

There is no single magic food that will prevent cognitive decline or guarantee longevity. But knowing how much is riding on a strong performance by your heart and blood vessels, you can identify which foods are particularly valuable in promoting brain health and overall wellness. Make sure you always have them on hand.

- ❑ **Green, leafy vegetables.** Kale, spinach, Swiss chard, and other greens are loaded with critical nutrients like vitamin K, which helps make proteins needed for the building of bones, and beta carotene, which converts into vitamin A and then plays an important role in cell growth and maintaining the health of the heart, lungs, and kidneys.
- ❑ **Fatty fish.** Salmon, mackerel, and sardines are known for their high concentrations of omega-3 fatty acids, which promote cardiovascular health and may lower your risk of stroke.
- ❑ **Tea and coffee.** Research has shown a statistical correlation between caffeine consumption and better memory.
- ❑ **Berries.** Packed with antioxidants that help fight free radicals and reduce oxidative stress in the body, these fruits also contain high levels of fiber, vitamins, and minerals, making them excellent allies in preventing chronic conditions like heart disease, diabetes, and cancer.
- ❑ **Beans.** Based on his experience studying the Blue Zones, Dan Buettner has nicknamed beans "the World's #1 Longevity Food." They're full of insoluble fiber, which promotes good bacteria in the gut, and they're high in protein, vitamins, and minerals.

And here's a roundup of some of our go-to herbs and spices, which not only add flavor to meals but double as nutritional powerhouses:

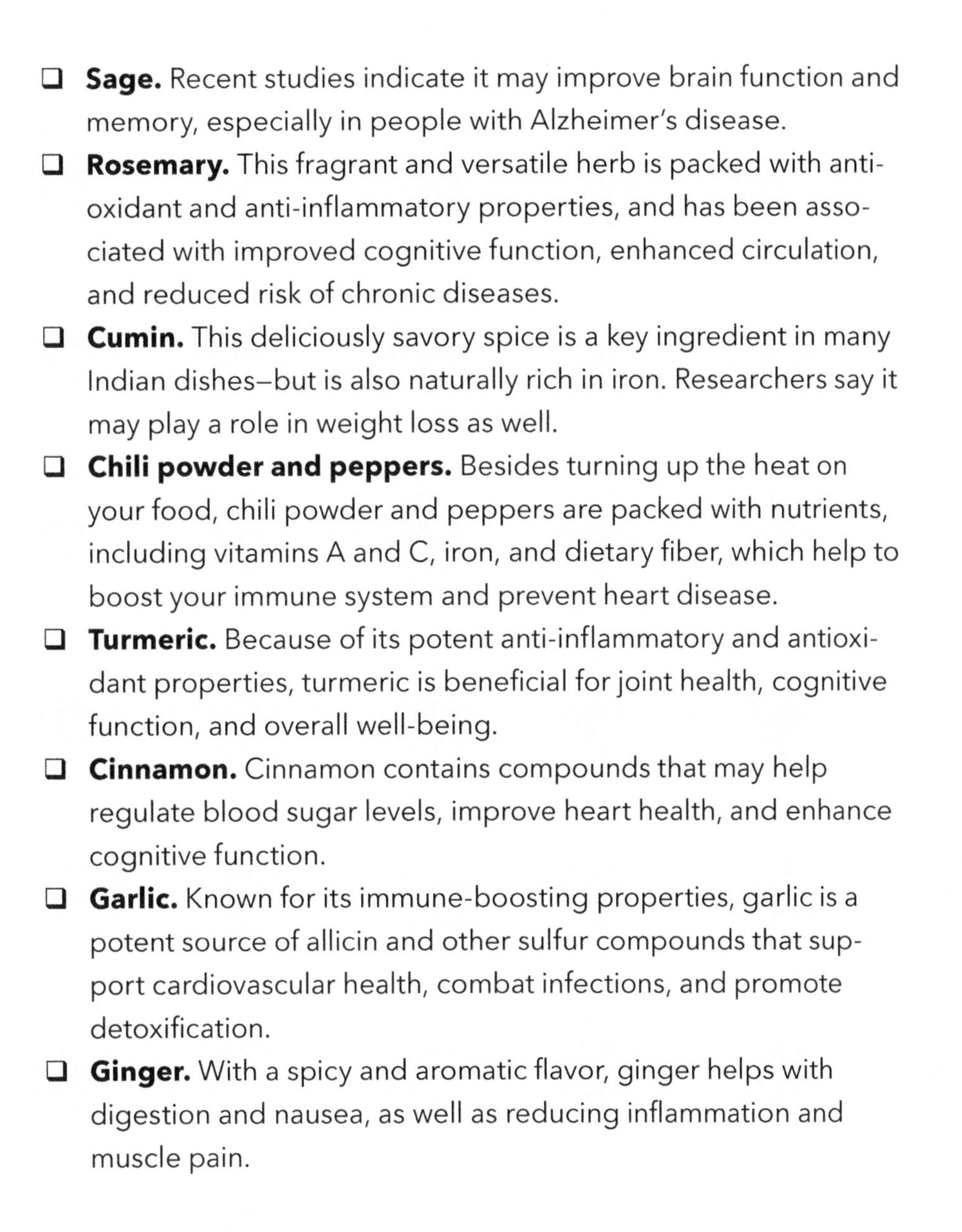

- ❑ **Sage.** Recent studies indicate it may improve brain function and memory, especially in people with Alzheimer's disease.
- ❑ **Rosemary.** This fragrant and versatile herb is packed with antioxidant and anti-inflammatory properties, and has been associated with improved cognitive function, enhanced circulation, and reduced risk of chronic diseases.
- ❑ **Cumin.** This deliciously savory spice is a key ingredient in many Indian dishes—but is also naturally rich in iron. Researchers say it may play a role in weight loss as well.
- ❑ **Chili powder and peppers.** Besides turning up the heat on your food, chili powder and peppers are packed with nutrients, including vitamins A and C, iron, and dietary fiber, which help to boost your immune system and prevent heart disease.
- ❑ **Turmeric.** Because of its potent anti-inflammatory and antioxidant properties, turmeric is beneficial for joint health, cognitive function, and overall well-being.
- ❑ **Cinnamon.** Cinnamon contains compounds that may help regulate blood sugar levels, improve heart health, and enhance cognitive function.
- ❑ **Garlic.** Known for its immune-boosting properties, garlic is a potent source of allicin and other sulfur compounds that support cardiovascular health, combat infections, and promote detoxification.
- ❑ **Ginger.** With a spicy and aromatic flavor, ginger helps with digestion and nausea, as well as reducing inflammation and muscle pain.

MAKE YOUR GROCERY LIST

Write down your SuperAging staples, then take a photo with your phone so that you always have your list available.

While fresh herbs often give a more vibrant flavor and aroma, dried spices offer convenience and versatility, especially when fresh ingredients are not readily available. Both dried spices and fresh herbs offer nutritional benefits, such as essential vitamins, minerals, and phytochemicals.

In general, dried herbs can retain their flavor and nutritional content for about one to three years when stored properly. To maximize their longevity, place in airtight containers such as glass jars or resealable bags, which prevent exposure to moisture. Dried herbs generally do better in a cool, dark place, such as a pantry or cupboard, away from direct sunlight and heat sources like stoves or ovens. Buying in bulk? They can also be frozen to extend their shelf life.

MAKE FITNESS AND EXERCISE PART OF YOUR SUPERAGING PROGRAM

- ❑ **Walk, strength train, squat.** Keep it simple. You don't need a gym or personal trainer. You can incorporate exercise into a convenient daily routine.
- ❑ **Strengthen your core.** A strong core helps improve balance and prevent falls, which are a major public health issue for the older population.
- ❑ **Improve your flexibility.** Regular stretching can improve your circulation, reduce your risk of joint and muscle pain, help you relax, and increase that range of motion (making all your other exercises more effective).
- ❑ **Practice good sleep habits.** Sleep deprivation produces many harmful effects on all ages, but there are particular implications for older people, including a connection between sleep problems and increased risk for dementia. Aim for at least seven hours per night. We mention the importance of sleep a lot, because it's fundamental to SuperAging and good health.
- ❑ **Consider team sports.** Team sports create a social network and reduce feelings of loneliness. They also enhance self-esteem and create an emotionally satisfying set of goals (teamwork, competitions) that contribute to better mental health.
- ❑ **Learn about exercise snacks.** Each exercise snack is typically only a few minutes long, and most snackers do it at least four or five times a day.
- ❑ **Know your numbers.** Fitness trackers and other wearables are now capable of capturing a huge range of data, including heart rate, sleep patterns, and calorie intake.

MISTAKES TO AVOID

We hear a lot about what to do when it comes to fitness, but not much about what we shouldn't do as SuperAgers. So we've included some mistakes to avoid when working out:

1. *Not drinking enough water.* Stay hydrated! Aim for at least eight glasses of eight ounces per day.
2. *Not warming up.* Stretch or do some other gentle warm-up before beginning your actual workout.
3. *Not modifying when necessary.* "TikTok tendonitis" is real, so be careful about doing an exercise routine you found on social media.
4. *Not breaking up long sessions into short bursts.* Short sessions of exercise have proved to be as effective as long exercise sessions.
5. *Not taking it slow.* We often think we can pick up right where we left off, but that's not always the case, especially if you haven't exercised in a while. Go slow.

One additional point needs to be made: As with anything involving exercise, make sure you've talked it over with your physician.

TAKE THE BALANCE TEST

Researchers at the Exercise Medicine Clinic in Rio de Janeiro used data from an exercise study that looked at the connection between ill health, death, and measures of physical fitness and exercise and concluded that the 10-second balance test should become part of routine health checks for all middle-aged and older adults. After taking into account differences in age, sex, and underlying health conditions, those who failed the balance test had an 84% higher risk of death from any cause in the subsequent decade.

Here's how to do it:

Stand on one foot (use either foot). Place the front of your free foot around the back of the foot that's on the floor. Hold your arms to the sides and look straight ahead. Hold the position for 10 seconds. If you can't do it at first, give yourself three tries.

TRACK YOUR EXERCISE

Use the pages that follow to track your progress for four weeks, develop your ideal workout schedule, and make fitness a permanent part of your SuperAging program.

DAY	EXERCISES	MUSCLE GROUPS	DURATION/ REPS	WEIGHTS	NOTES
MON					
TUE					
WED					
THU					
FRI					
SAT					
SUN					

Observations:

Modifications:

DAY	EXERCISES	MUSCLE GROUPS	DURATION/ REPS	WEIGHTS	NOTES
MON					
TUE					
WED					
THU					
FRI					
SAT					
SUN					

Observations:

Modifications:

DAY	EXERCISES	MUSCLE GROUPS	DURATION/ REPS	WEIGHTS	NOTES
MON					
TUE					
WED					
THU					
FRI					
SAT					
SUN					

Observations:

Modifications:

DAY	EXERCISES	MUSCLE GROUPS	DURATION/ REPS	WEIGHTS	NOTES
MON					
TUE					
WED					
THU					
FRI					
SAT					
SUN					

Observations:

Modifications:

MAKE BRAIN HEALTH PART OF YOUR SUPERAGING PROGRAM

- ❑ **Try new things.** The key is to offer variety to your brain. Many people gravitate to brain games and puzzles, but it's important not to limit yourself to things you've already mastered. You can keep doing those things for pure recreational enjoyment, of course, but, for better brain health, also tackle new types of puzzles or games that you're not familiar with.
- ❑ **Cultivate a hobby.** A 2022 study found that people with hobbies had fewer symptoms of depression as well as an enhanced sense of life satisfaction and happiness. In addition, hobbies can enhance social skills (Attachment), boost brain function (Activity), and improve fine motor skills (Activity).
- ❑ **Sleep well.** There is a connection between lack of sleep and heightened risk for dementia. One study showed that compared to people getting seven hours' sleep, people getting fewer hours each night are 30% more likely to be diagnosed with dementia. Whatever the underlying causes, it's clear that sleep deprivation increases your risk and better sleep reduces it. Aim for a minimum of seven hours per night.
- ❑ **Be aware of brain foods.** As discussed on pages 64–65, what you put on your plate can have a big impact on brain function. Stock up on the good stuff.
- ❑ **Understand how physical activity helps the brain.** Physical activity promotes increased oxygen flow and the growth of new nerve cells and synapses in the brain. It also lowers blood pressure and reduces stress, both of which are negative factors that increase the risk of dementia.
- ❑ **Nurture social connections.** Loneliness and social isolation increase the risk of dementia. So nurturing social connections becomes a big issue in the promotion of brain health. It's such an important topic, in fact, that it makes up one of our seven *A*'s of SuperAging (see p. 132).

CULTIVATE A HOBBY

Do you have any hobbies? Despite the aforementioned benefits, many adults are reluctant to pick up a hobby. They may be afraid of failing or looking silly, or they might simply feel like spending time on a pleasurable activity is a waste. But starting a new hobby ticks off two items from our list of ways to make brain health part of your SuperAging program.

Here are some tips and exercises to help you overcome your hesitation and get started on cultivating a hobby.

- [ ] **Start small.** Too often when we hear "new hobby," we think about all the time and effort it will take to get halfway decent. Focus instead on the fun, and start small. Rather than your goal being to become fluent in a new language, for example, learn how to order a coffee.

What's a quick activity you could try?

- [ ] **Reflect on your childhood.** What did you love to do when you were a kid? Is there a grown-up version you could try?

What were your favorite things to do as a child?

FIGURE SKATER AT 53

After a 37-year hiatus, Didi Gluck rediscovered a love of figure skating in her early 50s. She'd quit the sport in high school, following a childhood spent pushing herself and competing. But, motivated by a friend, Gluck started skating again in adulthood and discovered a healthier attitude toward the sport and toward herself. She's even returned to competitions.

- ❑ **Consider moments when you've been "in the zone."** Also known as "flow state," being in the zone means you've lost track of time and performance anxiety. Instead, you're fully immersed in the task at hand. Thinking about times when you've been in the zone can help point you toward a meaningful hobby.

When have you been in the zone?

INVENTOR AT 66

After watching his wife, Betsey, struggle to peel vegetables due to her arthritis, Sam Farber developed a line of inclusive kitchen tools, OXO. He was 66 and had already retired from a successful career in kitchenware when inspiration struck. OXO's innovation was a special handle designed to be comfortable and easy to hold, regardless of grip strength or hand size.

WHAT'S STOPPING YOU?

Consider some hobbies that interest you or that you've always wanted to check out. Make a list of what's preventing you from giving them a try. The idea of this activity isn't to focus on the negatives, but to see whether there are creative solutions to perceived challenges. For instance, maybe you'd like to try pickleball, but you're hesitant about investing in expensive equipment. Is there a friend or neighbor who has a racket you can borrow for the day? Can you find a class at a community center where you can try it out?

POTENTIAL HOBBY	CHALLENGE	SOLUTION

KEY TAKEAWAYS

Use this space to write down your key takeaways, notes to self, and anything else you'd like to remember from this chapter.

NEXT STEPS

Remember the honorary eighth pillar: *Accountability.* Fill in the blanks, giving yourself a reasonable time horizon. Be as specific as possible about the action and your reason(s) for undertaking it. Concrete whys help ensure follow-through.

In the next ____________, I will ____.

I'm going to do this because ____.

I'm also excited to ____.

READ MORE

There is a direct correlation between reading and other factors or influences that promote longevity. For example, a 2013 study that carried out brain scans while participants were reading a novel over a course of time showed that the reading increased brain connectivity. Reading also gradually helped participants develop larger vocabularies and increased the ability of readers to understand others' feelings. Brain activity and emotional connection to others are two hallmarks of longevity.

CHAPTER 5

ACCOMPLISHMENT

YOUR ACCOMPLISHMENTS DON'T END WITH RETIREMENT

In the context of SuperAging, Accomplishment means viewing the post-65 phase of life not as a period of retreat and disengagement but as an extended and positive opportunity to continue to grow and achieve goals.

SuperAging areas of Accomplishment include:

- Employment and un-retirement (returning to the workforce after you've retired)
- Volunteering and other unpaid opportunities
- Education, including online learning

MAKE ACCOMPLISHMENT PART OF YOUR SUPERAGING PROGRAM

In this section, you will learn how to:

- ❑ **Define a goal or purpose.** It is almost impossible to overstate the importance of laying out a purpose and specific goals for accomplishment. What have you always wanted to do but didn't have time for? What area of your life would you like to improve?
- ❑ **Research the categories of possibility.** SuperAgers envision the post-65 period of life as a time of continuing to set and achieve goals. Start thinking about other types of employment or volunteering you might be interested in trying. Consider the things you do that make you feel "in the zone." (See p. 77 in chapter 4, Activity.)
- ❑ **Consider a life or retirement coach.** Experts in this rapidly growing field offer specific advice on "what to do with the rest of your life," based on the specifics of the individual clients–their age, their position (employed / near retirement / retired) as well as their interests and goals.

DEFINE YOUR PURPOSE AND GOALS

People with a sense of purpose (and the optimism that they can/will achieve that purpose) actually live longer than people without that sense of purpose.

We're not talking here about a vague "feel-good" mood. We're talking about specifics: *Put it in writing.* What do you want to accomplish over the next year? The next five years? Ten? Twenty? Your goals may be occupation-oriented, or they may be focused on things like maintaining relationships (Attachment) and aging in place (Autonomy), both of which we cover in coming chapters.

In the next year, I want to:

To accomplish that goal, I plan to:

In the next five years, I want to:

To accomplish that goal, I plan to:

In the next 10 years, I want to:

To accomplish that goal, I plan to:

In the next 20 years, I want to:

To accomplish that goal, I plan to:

BEST-SELLING AUTHOR AT 65

Laura Ingalls Wilder began writing her beloved *Little House on the Prairie* books in her 60s. Her stories, based on her childhood experiences, became classics in American literature. The first book was published when she was 65, and the series has since been adapted into numerous TV shows and movies, inspiring generations of readers.

TAKE THE GREAT REASSESSMENT QUIZ BY LISA DA ROCHA

Toronto-based life coach Lisa Da Rocha developed this quiz to help you figure out where you are with your life and career goals. Da Rocha's quiz offers two significant lessons for SuperAgers. On the one hand, it's important to understand where you're coming from—that is, which attitudes, likes, needs, and desires you are bringing to the situation.

On the other hand, even as you're (quite rightly) accumulating information about what the next stages might entail, and where the best opportunities might lie, it's important not to overthink things, especially at the outset. Don't let your information-gathering and analysis go too far too quickly and block you from testing and experimentation. Take the following quiz, checking which option you align with most.

My life and career have purpose and meaning that is important to me.	*Strongly disagree*	*Disagree*	*Agree*	*Strongly agree*
I feel that my talents are well utilized and appreciated.	*Strongly disagree*	*Disagree*	*Agree*	*Strongly agree*
I've defined what a "life well lived" looks like for me and invest my time and effort in these areas.	*Strongly disagree*	*Disagree*	*Agree*	*Strongly agree*
There's something in my life, beyond myself, that I am contributing to.	*Strongly disagree*	*Disagree*	*Agree*	*Strongly agree*
I believe that with focus and energy I can create, learn, and develop anything.	*Strongly disagree*	*Disagree*	*Agree*	*Strongly agree*
My work and life offer me plenty of opportunities to learn and grow.	*Strongly disagree*	*Disagree*	*Agree*	*Strongly agree*
I have hobbies, activities, and/or people in my life that expand and stretch me.	*Strongly disagree*	*Disagree*	*Agree*	*Strongly agree*
I embrace the fact that I am both a work in progress and perfect as I am.	*Strongly disagree*	*Disagree*	*Agree*	*Strongly agree*
I get seven to nine hours of sleep every night.	*Never*	*Sometimes*	*Most of the time*	*Always*
I eat a healthy, nutritious whole-food diet.	*Never*	*Sometimes*	*Most of the time*	*Always*

I get 30 minutes of moderate exercise every day (e.g., walking).	*Never*	*Sometimes*	*Most of the time*	*Always*
I use strategies that help me manage stress effectively.	*Strongly disagree*	*Disagree*	*Agree*	*Strongly agree*
I can balance the positive and negative aspects of any situation, circumstance, and person.	*Strongly disagree*	*Disagree*	*Agree*	*Strongly agree*
I can accept all my emotions without getting caught up in the story or being right.	*Strongly disagree*	*Disagree*	*Agree*	*Strongly agree*
I have deep, supportive, and positive relationships in my life.	*Strongly disagree*	*Disagree*	*Agree*	*Strongly agree*
I feel comfortable asking others for help.	*Strongly disagree*	*Disagree*	*Agree*	*Strongly agree*
I feel connected and supported by my coworkers.	*Strongly disagree*	*Disagree*	*Agree*	*Strongly agree*
I invest quality time in building deep relationships with people who are important to me.	*Strongly disagree*	*Disagree*	*Agree*	*Strongly agree*
I engage in activities outside of work that bring me joy.	*Strongly disagree*	*Disagree*	*Agree*	*Strongly agree*
I have things in my life that I am excited about.	*Strongly disagree*	*Disagree*	*Agree*	*Strongly agree*
I maximize my energy by honoring rest and renewal.	*Strongly disagree*	*Disagree*	*Agree*	*Strongly agree*
I create a life of play and laughter.	*Strongly disagree*	*Disagree*	*Agree*	*Strongly agree*

The scoring is straightforward. You'll notice that the choices run in a continuum, left to right, from negative ("Strongly disagree" / "Never") to positive ("Strongly agree" / "Always").

Score 1 point for every time you chose the first option offered (extreme left) and 2 points for the next one over, 3 points for the next, working up to 4 points for every answer that was the most positive (extreme right). The highest-possible score is 88.

YOUR SCORE: ____________________

The test is intended as a self-audit—there are no "right" or "wrong" answers—but Da Rocha did develop some useful descriptors of an individual's "state of play," depending on their final total. We found both the categories and the descriptions to be interesting and helpful:

Score of 70–80: CREATED LIFE. You've defined what is important to you, and your actions are aligned with these things. CONGRATULATIONS! You are creating your life.

Score of 50–70: INTENTIONAL LIFE. You're making great progress and spending most of your time and effort on the things and people that are a priority for you. You are living with intention.

Score of 30–50: CONSCIOUS LIFE. You are conscious of what is working and not working and have taken some small steps in making changes. This is where a lot of people get discouraged because you've been working hard for a while, but living a life that is fulfilling and exciting still feels far off. Do not give up! You're doing the right things, and it's important to persevere.

Score of 15–30: DEFINED LIFE. You've started to think about what is most important to you and how you want things to change. You are beginning to see where in your life you are living to please others, rather than yourself. You've been experimenting and seeing what works for you. Now is the time to fully commit and determine where you want to focus and what support you need along the way.

Score of 0–15: DEFAULT LIFE. You're in the early phases of defining what is important to you and how you might create a life and career that is aligned to your unique vision of success. Your life may feel overwhelming and frustrating at times, but concentrate on small wins and keep moving forward.

Spend a few minutes reflecting on your score. What did this quiz teach you about yourself?

SET YOURSELF A WEEK OF DAILY CHALLENGES

Sometimes, when we think about Accomplishment, we get fixated on huge goals like earning a degree or starting a business. But Accomplishment can occur on a much smaller scale, and these small wins can motivate you toward setting and accomplishing a larger goal.

Spend a week setting yourself daily challenges. Again, these challenges can be small, such as syncing your smartphone with your smart home devices, updating your LinkedIn page or website, or researching volunteering opportunities.

Monday's challenge:

Did you accomplish it? Y / N

Next steps or follow-up:

Tuesday's challenge:

Did you accomplish it? Y / N

Next steps or follow-up:

Wednesday's challenge:

Did you accomplish it? Y / N

Next steps or follow-up:

Thursday's challenge:

Did you accomplish it? Y / N

Next steps or follow-up:

Friday's challenge:

Did you accomplish it? Y / N

Next steps or follow-up:

Saturday's challenge:

Did you accomplish it? Y / N

Next steps or follow-up:

Sunday's challenge:

Did you accomplish it? Y / N

Next steps or follow-up:

TAKE THE RETIREMENT READINESS QUIZ BY JOHN WINDSOR

The practice of lifestyle coach John Windsor is geared toward people specifically engaged with the retirement topic. So his questions cover not only attitude but "readiness"—emotional, social, financial, and more. Again, there are no "right" and "wrong" answers; the value lies in provoking your awareness of the topics and the current state of both your attitude and your circumstances.

How do you feel about retirement?

❑ I can't wait
❑ I can't retire
❑ I feel a mix of excitement and dread
❑ I'm not interested in a typical retirement

When do you intend to retire?

❑ It's coming soon
❑ In the next three to five years
❑ I have no idea
❑ I'm not going to retire
❑ I can't

What plans do you have for this new phase in your life?

❑ I have a long list of projects and activities I want to tackle
❑ No major plans, except to sleep in and see what tomorrow brings
❑ I want to keep doing "something," whether or not it's called work
❑ I have some ideas of things to do, but a plan is not fully formed yet

How's your health?

❑ It's okay, I think
❑ It's great; I could live to 105
❑ I have health issues

How important is fitness to you?

❑ It's not something I think about a lot
❑ Getting regular walks each week works for me
❑ I do something almost every day

How long do you think you'll live?
- ❑ At least into my 90s
- ❑ I hope to get to 80 or so
- ❑ I never think about it

What will you do for fun during retirement?
- ❑ I have no clue
- ❑ The possibilities are endless
- ❑ I'll figure it out; I'm good at finding fun things to do
- ❑ I have a few things on my list

How important is having a sense of purpose in what you do?
- ❑ I just want to enjoy each day without any commitments
- ❑ Sounds great, but I'm not sure what that would be
- ❑ This is really important, and I have a clear idea of how I want to contribute

How will your identity change when you retire?
- ❑ It won't change; I am who I am
- ❑ There's going to be a period of transition to deal with
- ❑ This is something I'm concerned about
- ❑ I don't know
- ❑ I have no idea what you're talking about

What fears do you have about your retirement?
- ❑ Running out of money
- ❑ Being bored
- ❑ I have no fears about it
- ❑ I feel anxious about it, but I'm not sure why
- ❑ That something will happen that will affect my ability to work

Do you have a spouse or significant other?
- ❑ Yes
- ❑ That's not a factor for me
- ❑ No

What does this person think about your plans?
- ❑ Totally on board with whatever I decide
- ❑ Not enthused about what may happen
- ❑ This is an ongoing topic of discussion
- ❑ Not applicable

Where will you live during this next phase of your life? ❑ I haven't thought that much about it ❑ I don't want to move ❑ I can't move ❑ I'm going to move ❑ I'll let my other plans dictate where I live
How do you feel about "change" in your life? ❑ I'm not a fan, unless I can be in control ❑ I embrace it, even when it's hard ❑ It's part of life; you deal with it
How involved will you be with family during retirement? ❑ We'll get together from time to time ❑ I'll see them as much as possible ❑ We're not really connected
What kind of social network do you have? ❑ I have lots of friends, near and far ❑ I have a handful of close friends, but not all are nearby ❑ I don't have many people that I am in regular contact with
How prepared are you financially for this next chapter in your life? ❑ Super prepared; I could last 30 years or more without working ❑ I'm partway there but can't stop working yet ❑ I don't want to stop making money or working ❑ I can never retire ❑ I don't know
Have you developed a budget or financial plan for your future? ❑ No ❑ Yes; I did it myself ❑ Yes; I worked with a financial planner
How important is it to leave a legacy? ❑ It's a nice concept, but I'm not thinking about it ❑ This is really important to me; I want to know that I mattered ❑ I like to be helpful; I think that's enough
How old are you? ❑ Under 55 ❑ 55–64 ❑ 65-plus

There's no scoring involved with this quiz. Instead, each question gives you a chance to reflect on your current circumstances and state of mind as they relate to retirement. Write down your thoughts and observations below. What did this quiz teach you about yourself?

Based on your answers and self-reflection, are you ready to retire? Why or why not?

RESEARCH THE CATEGORIES OF POSSIBILITY

As you think about life after retirement, get to know the full spectrum of possibilities and resources that are out there. You may certainly concentrate your Accomplishment goals based on your personal preferences; you should not, however, limit them because you don't know what's possible and available.

We recommend organizing your research into three logical categories—Paid Employment, Unpaid Employment, and Education and Self-Improvement—and assembling information using the techniques we outlined in the "Awareness" chapter. Each category in turn sets up logical subcategories and offers a rich and ambitious menu of choices. Use your results from the previous quizzes to gain insight into what might be right for you in the years to come.

> As reported by human resources consultant Mercer, people over the age of 75 "will constitute the fastest-growing age band in the civilian workforce between now and 2030." In fact, according to CNN, this age group has more than quadrupled in size since 1964, and it's expected that the cohort of older working Americans will double over the next 10 years.

EMPLOYMENT

When it comes to employment, we envision a few possible avenues, both paid and unpaid.

PAID EMPLOYMENT

- Continue with current job full time
- Continue with current job part time
- New full-time job, including returning to the workforce
- New part-time job or gig
- Buy or open a new business

Thinking about your present situation and future goals, which of these options (if any) feels right to you?

PRESIDENT AND FOUNDER OF A BIOTECH COMPANY AT 70+

Throughout his career, Dr. Robert Young has helped design and synthesize many life-changing drugs, including treatments for osteoporosis, asthma, and arthritis. Following his retirement from a major pharmaceutical company, he founded—and continues to serve as president of—a biotech start-up that's pioneering new drugs and drug delivery systems.

UNPAID EMPLOYMENT

You might wish to commit to nonmonetary employment, now or in the future. For example, you could:

- Volunteer for a local organization
- Pursue an overseas volunteer opportunity
- Become a mentor or go after a similar opportunity

Thinking about your present situation and future goals, which of these options (if any) feels right to you?

EDUCATION AND SELF-IMPROVEMENT

When it comes to education, no matter what you're looking for, you will find an institution and a program to suit your needs and wants. For example, you could:

- Take for-credit courses leading to credentials (e.g., degree, diploma, certification)
- Take not-for-credit courses at universities and colleges
- Try online learning, whether for-credit or not-for-credit
- Become a personal coach, trainer, or teacher of new skills

Thinking about your present situation and future goals, which of these options (if any) feels right to you?

A 2020 paper published in *American Economic Review* found that entrepreneurs over 50 were almost twice as likely to be successful as those in their 30s, with age being an often-overlooked factor in their success. Older entrepreneurs tend to be more financially stable and have bigger networks, with a set of strong, transferable skills.

Use the chart below to make **paid employment** part of your Awareness routine.

PAID EMPLOYMENT	SOURCES	
Subtopics or areas of interest	Books	Newspapers, magazines

Key search terms for intermittent sources related to paid employment:

Use the chart below to make **unpaid employment** part of your Awareness routine.

UNPAID EMPLOYMENT	SOURCES	
Subtopics or areas of interest	Books	Newspapers, magazines

Key search terms for intermittent sources related to unpaid employment:

SOURCES (PAID EMPLOYMENT)			
Websites, e-newsletters	Videos, podcasts	Apps	Other

SOURCES (UNPAID EMPLOYMENT)			
Websites, e-newsletters	Videos, podcasts	Apps	Other

Use the chart below to make **education and self-improvement** part of your Awareness routine.

EDUCATION & SELF-IMPROVEMENT	SOURCES	
Subtopics or areas of interest	Books	Newspapers, magazines

Key search terms for intermittent sources related to education and self-improvement:

PHD AT 89

Following a successful career as a medical doctor and professor of hematology, Manfred Steiner fulfilled a lifelong dream of earning a PhD in physics. He was 89. Growing up during World War II, Dr. Steiner opted for what his family considered to be a more practical route into medicine, rather than pursuing the sciences. He started taking classes after his retirement from academic medicine, eventually earning enough credits for a doctorate from Brown University.

SOURCES (EDUCATION & SELF-IMPROVEMENT)			
Websites, e-newsletters	Videos, podcasts	Apps	Other

HUMANITARIAN ARCHITECT AT 59

In 1964, at age 23, Yasmeen Lari became the first female architect in Pakistan. After she retired from commercial work in 2000, she embarked on an "encore career" focused on creating low-cost, environmentally friendly homes for marginalized and rural populations, including victims of natural disasters. Some 50,000 low-cost shelters have been constructed thus far.

WHAT WILL YOU DO FOR FUN?

The wording may be casual, even throwaway, but the underlying idea behind this question speaks to a major aspect of SuperAging that is too easy to overlook. SuperAging means having a good time! Yes, it's a revolution in the whole concept of aging and, yes, it involves significant activities and achievements that transform the individual life as well as society as a whole. Big, meaningful stuff, in other words. But SuperAgers also want to have a lot of fun along the way. While SuperAging definitely includes growth and achievement, these shouldn't be seen as burdens. They aren't mandatory expectations imposed from some external pressure to live up to an intense new model.

With these insights in mind, ask yourself, *What will I do for fun?* List or write out your answers.

Today:

In coming years:

DESCRIBE YOUR DREAM LIFE

Be as detailed as possible. What does your dream life look like?

WHAT'S ON YOUR BUCKET LIST?

Even if you haven't seen the 2007 movie, you likely know what a bucket list is: basically, a list of things you want to do before you die. Having one indicates at least some foundational belief in the possibility of checking off many, if not all, of the items.

Your bucket list should include things you're passionate about and interested in. If you're having trouble listing things, consider focusing on a category, such as national parks you want to visit or bands you'd like to see in concert.

TRY NEW THINGS

We mentioned the importance of trying new things several times in the context of keeping your brain healthy. But trying new things can also be a low-stakes way of anticipating a new and exciting future.

Make a list of new things you'd like to try. Once again, simple is best—taking an Italian cooking class, for example, or exploring a state park near your house. Bookmark or put a sticky note on this page so you can refer back to it as you try different things and expand your initial list.

TRACK YOUR ACTIVITIES

Use this chart to keep track of your favorite new activities and experiences. Over time, you may discover a whole new avenue of hobbies, interests, skills, employment, or other areas of Accomplishment.

ACTIVITY	THOUGHTS & OBSERVATIONS	WOULD YOU DO IT AGAIN?

WHAT'S BLOCKING YOU?

In her practice, life coach Lisa Da Rocha found that the very skills that made her clients successful can, paradoxically, block a transition to the next phase. Those skills typically include strong analytical and problem-solving abilities, a very well-organized work ethic, consciousness of deadlines, and good time allocation. In sum: a strong left brain. What's blocking you? List any attitudes, characteristics, or beliefs that might be preventing you from going after a goal.

KEY TAKEAWAYS

Use this space to write down your key takeaways, notes to self, and anything else you'd like to remember from this chapter.

NEXT STEPS

Remember the honorary eighth pillar: *Accountability.* Fill in the blanks, giving yourself a reasonable time horizon. Be as specific as possible about the action and your reason(s) for undertaking it. Concrete whys help ensure follow-through.

In the next ______________, I will ______________________________
______________________________.

I'm going to do this because ______________________________
______________________________.

I'm also excited to ______________________________
______________________________.

ASTRONAUT AT 90

Actor William Shatner became the oldest person in space when he traveled aboard a privately owned spacecraft in 2021. He was 90 when he crossed the Kármán line, generally considered to be the boundary between the atmosphere and space, approximately 63 miles above Earth. Shatner is best known for playing fictional starship captain James T. Kirk in the Star Trek franchise.

CHAPTER 6

AUTONOMY

AUTONOMY TAKES PLANNING

Both DefaultAgers and SuperAgers want to live independently for as long as possible, of course. But SuperAgers don't leave such a future up to chance. Instead, they focus on three main areas:

1. Housing
2. Healthcare
3. Money

SuperAgers see the home as an active provider of autonomy. In addition to ensuring lifestyle-enhancing amenities, SuperAgers see the home as an ever-more-important locus of healthcare. And, thanks to heightened Awareness, SuperAgers take a much more active role in managing both their health and their money.

MAKE AUTONOMY PART OF YOUR SUPERAGING PROGRAM

In this section, you will learn how to:

- ❑ **Start thinking about Autonomy every day.**
- ❑ **Conduct an Autonomy audit of your current living space.**
- ❑ **Evaluate your existing doctor and financial adviser.**
- ❑ **Build Awareness around age-tech and healthcare.**

CONDUCT AN AUTONOMY AUDIT

Unless you have some reason to already be planning to sell your home and move, unconnected with any SuperAging issues, you should assume you will age in place and conduct a formal Autonomy audit. The audit will reveal weaknesses and the kind of action (and cost) that will be needed to improve your home's ability to support your Autonomy over the long term.

You may want to conduct this audit on your own through a simple checklist (which we offer here) or engage a professional. As with the financial planning sector, the construction renovation sector is actively training and certifying specialists in home renovation for aging in place.

Why do an audit now? This is really an extension of our first recommendation: Start paying attention to the topic and the issues. Even if it's just a dry-run exercise and you may be years away from taking action, it will help you consider the range of home features that you may be taking for granted.

	Y / N	NOTES	NEXT STEPS
		EXTERIOR	
Adequate lighting			
No-step entry			
Wider doorways			
Lever-style door handles			
Space for a ramp			
Driveway			
Front walkway			
Lawn/garden			
Pool			
		OVERALL (THROUGHOUT YOUR HOME)	
Adequate lighting			
Wider doorways			
Lever-style door handles			
Carpet or rugs			
		BATHROOM	
Higher toilet height			
Grab bars for toilet and bath/shower			
Walk-in shower/tub			
Handheld showerhead			
Slip-resistant floors			

	Y / N	NOTES	NEXT STEPS
KITCHEN			
Sink height			
Hands-free faucet			
Larger drawers			
Pull-out pantry			
Cabinets lower, more accessible			
Pull-down shelves			
BEDROOM			
Location (near a bathroom? Ground floor or upstairs?)			
Lighting in the closet			
Bed rail			
LAUNDRY ROOM			
Location (near a bedroom? Ground floor or in the basement?)			
Front-load appliances			
Appliances raised 12–15 inches			
Cabinets lower, more accessible			
Pull-down shelves			

It's easy to see how our suggestions relate to possible future physical issues. Hands-free faucets if arthritis makes it harder to turn taps; ramps and stair lifts for easier mobility; wider doorways if a walker or wheelchair is involved.

If these needs are imminent, we strongly recommend hiring a professional with specific experience (and, ideally, credentials) in serving the aging-in-place market. If you're just doing an early practice run, it's enough to start looking at your home through the lens of what Autonomy will require down the road.

HELP YOURSELF AGE IN PLACE

Based on your home audit, what happens next? Do you hire a contractor? Do you make nonpermanent modifications? Do you look for a new space? What's your timeline?

DECLUTTER

Clutter has been shown to increase anxiety and decrease productivity. It also makes it hard to clean and difficult to age in place.

Regardless of your situation—whether you're moving to a new space or modifying the space you're in, or simply want to get organized—you can use our decluttering checklist to corral your stuff.

1. Begin by going through your space and determining which areas are most in need of decluttering. Write down your plan, including the order in which you plan to tackle your rooms, as well as your time frame:

2. Label four boxes: Keep, Donate, Maybe, and Trash. If you're undecided about what to do with an item, stick it in the Maybe box. Delaying the decision about what to do can help give you clarity—just make sure you eventually decide, and don't wind up with another box full of clutter.
3. Designate an area to store your boxes so that it doesn't feel like you're creating clutter or a mess while decluttering.
4. Utilize our room-by-room guide on the next page.
5. Reorganize your space, finding new spots for anything in the Keep box as necessary.
6. Deal with the remaining boxes, including making final decisions around the Maybe box, and enjoy your decluttered space!

TAKE DECLUTTERING ONE STEP AT A TIME

Follow these checklists to declutter your space room by room.

Bathroom

- ❑ Get rid of grooming products you no longer use. Makeup can expire, so be careful about hanging on to old items.
- ❑ Return old or expired medications to your local pharmacy, or put them in used coffee grounds or cat litter in the trash. Don't flush them! Many medicines contain chemicals that don't break down when you flush or pour them down the drain. These chemicals enter our water supply and can harm the ecosystem.

Bedroom

- ❑ Tackle the closet and bureaus, getting rid of clothes you no longer wear.
- ❑ Donate old jewelry. Consider your local thrift store or a "Buy Nothing" group on Facebook.
- ❑ Clean under the bed. An "out of sight, out of mind" approach can lead to chaos.
- ❑ Remove everything from the tops of nightstands and other flat services. Carefully and thoughtfully put things back.

SET A TIMER

Feeling overwhelmed? Set a timer. Aim to declutter for 15 minutes at a pop. When the timer goes off, you can stop for the day. You just might find, however, that you're able to go for longer once you get started.

- ❑ Create a system for keeping clothes off the floor, such as a hamper or attractive basket. If clothes tend to accumulate on a chair, remove the chair until you've broken the habit.
- ❑ Call a local animal shelter and see whether they might be willing to take bedding and blankets that you're not using. Otherwise, look for a textile recycling event (usually run by the sanitation department) near you.

Living Room

- ❑ Take everything off the shelves. The simple act of holding an item can often help you decide whether to keep, donate, or trash it.
- ❑ Be selective about collections—a few representative items artfully displayed can be more meaningful than shelf after shelf of collectibles.
- ❑ Donate unwanted books to your local library, religious organization, or thrift store. Some organizations like NYC Books Through Bars also facilitate book donations to prisons.
- ❑ Look for an e-waste event in your area to get rid of old cords, remote controls, monitors, phones, and any other obsolete electronics. Avoid throwing them into the trash, as electronics may contain hazardous waste. Contact your sanitation department for info about proper disposal.
- ❑ Freshen up your photos, swapping out older pics for newer ones. You'll be amazed at how new your space feels simply by changing out items you see every day.
- ❑ Avoid using your living room as a de facto storage space. Put items, such as shoes or handbags, back where they belong. Recycle magazines and newspapers after you've read them.

Kitchen

- ❑ Go one cabinet or drawer at a time, to avoid feeling overwhelmed.
- ❑ Remove everything from the refrigerator and freezer (and give them a good scrub!). Put foods back in an organized, accessible

way, including the fruit and vegetables in a spot where you'll see and use them.

- ❑ Check the expiration date of anything you want to put back into the cabinet, pantry, fridge, or freezer. Use this opportunity to restock with SuperAging foods (see p. 64).
- ❑ Throw away broken items.
- ❑ Recycle old menus, magazines, or recipes, and donate any cookbooks that you don't use or want.

MAINTAIN YOUR SYSTEM

Here's how to avoid backsliding into Clutterville:

- ❑ Spend a few minutes tidying up every day.
- ❑ Have a routine for things that tend to pile up, such as going through and sorting your mail every Sunday, or putting away your laundry as soon as it's folded.
- ❑ Avoid stockpiling items. A sale isn't so great when you don't have space for another 18 rolls of paper towels.

GIVE AWAY WITH CARE

We all have items we can't bear to see wind up in the trash. However, giving a once-prized possession to someone who doesn't want it is foisting clutter onto them. Ask before you give, and don't be offended if someone passes on the item. Their decision isn't a reflection of you, your taste, or your relationship.

PICK YOUR LONGEVITY TEAM

If you're the quarterback of your future (and SuperAgers definitely see themselves that way), these are the people who can form the protective pocket and help you move the ball. You may not need all of them all at once, but you should at least know who belongs on your longevity team and what they can do for you. Use the following list to start researching possible partners, and jot down their contact info below so you can get in touch.

- ❑ **Financial planner—but specially trained and certified.** There are now several certificates or other designations (such as CSA, or Certified Senior Advisor) that signify additional training and experience in longevity-related issues.
- ❑ **Geriatrician.** Specializing in elder care, a geriatrician can offer advice around medication, management of chronic conditions, and other issues related to health, wellness, and longevity.
- ❑ **Estate planning attorney.** An estate attorney specializes in wills and trusts, and in dealing with complex tax issues. They can also look at long-term health issues, power of attorney, living wills, and other related topics.
- ❑ **Specialist Realtor.** SuperAgers may face complex real estate issues. Do you cash out and downsize? And if so, where do you move to? What about a reverse mortgage and blended families? A specialist Realtor can talk with you about your options.
- ❑ **Insurance specialist.** Do you need supplemental insurance or long-term-care insurance? An insurance specialist will help you identify the right products for you.
- ❑ **Occupational therapist.** An OT can assess your current residence through the lens of what you'll need down the road to maintain your autonomy, advise on products and services, and develop a plan to get you there.
- ❑ **Life coach.** We predict that consulting with a retirement or reinvention coach will become as routine as seeing an expert on health and wellness or exercise or investments.

WHO'S ON YOUR LONGEVITY TEAM?

Start to research how you could go about creating your own Longevity Team. Are there resources or individuals in your area? What about recommendations from friends, family, or colleagues? Write down the results of your research, noting any follow-ups or next steps.

NAME AND CONTACT INFO	DATE CONTACTED	NOTES AND NEXT STEPS

EVALUATE YOUR DOCTOR

Here we're only talking about the GP or family physician, your first line of medical assessment and the gatekeeper to the entire system. We can't offer generalized advice about dealing with specialists who may be treating serious conditions. But, for the family physician, it is reasonable to undertake an audit of the doctor's knowledge and approach. Below are key questions to consider, along with space to write down your thoughts and experiences with your doctor.

What is the doctor's overall attitude? Is the doctor arrogant or condescending? There may have been a time when you needed to accept this; that time has passed.

Are they a good listener? If not, this could be a sign of ageism, as in: Your views don't matter, the doctor is in charge, let's just hurry things along.

Is each visit a separate and distinct event or part of a continuum? In DefaultAging, the transaction model prevailed. You got sick, you went to the doctor, you got better, you didn't see the doctor again until the next time you were sick. Is the doctor aware of your overall treatment history, or any patterns? Is your chart readily available on the doctor's computer screen? Do they ever act as if they're not 100% sure who you are?

How do they respond to your concerns? Is your doctor interested in or dismissive of information or ideas you yourself may be advancing? Are you afraid to bring up something you saw on the internet? Are you nervous about mentioning things like supplements or alternative therapies?

Are they aware of emerging new technologies for diagnostics and better patient service? Telehealth, wireless trackers, electronic health records, and other technology can make it easier for you to age at home. As you build awareness around age-tech, is your doctor following suit?

Do they have any idea about your future potential and your actual plans? This is another aspect of a one-shot transaction versus a continuum of care. Does your doctor think you are a SuperAger? Do they even know what that is? Have they ever shown any interest in what you might be up to in five or 10 years—and what the healthcare implications are for that goal? Or is it always just the immediate issue of today's visit?

If you were a customer instead of a patient, how would your doctor stack up? Do the appointments start on time? Is the facility clean and bright, the supporting staff friendly? Taking the whole package together as one, is it an enterprise that understands you and your needs, and that is motivated to deliver outstanding service? Thinking like a consumer, would you rather take your business elsewhere?

EVALUATE YOUR FINANCIAL ADVISER

When it comes to your financial adviser, you can get, if you want, a daily (or even hourly) readout of how you're doing, and you may well decide to put up with a certain degree of less-than-stellar service as long as the numbers remain good. So it's not for us to casually advise any individual SuperAger to fire their financial adviser!

The chances are good that a SuperAger's financial adviser has already proved themself, to some degree, over the years and in varying market conditions. But it still makes sense to conduct an audit (even if only a dialogue with yourself). What you're after here is not so much stock-picking ability, but breadth of knowledge about the many new financial challenges and opportunities generated by the SuperAging revolution. Does the adviser have a wide-enough horizon? You could form those judgments yourself, based on your experience with that financial adviser. We recommend asking the adviser some pointed questions like these, then jotting down their answers:

Are you aware of my future plans? Does it surprise your advisor to learn you might be planning to continue working past age 65?

How do you think that would influence the financial program we've developed together?

Are you aware of my current housing situation and its suitability/unsuitability for aging in place? Does your adviser think you can stay in your current home? Do they have an idea of changes or upgrades you should make, and what they would cost? Are they able to map out those costs over an extended period of time (perhaps decades)?

Do you think that knowledge about Autonomy and aging in place should be considered as part of your responsibilities?

How should I prepare to pay for healthcare? Some healthcare costs may be covered by government plans, some by private insurance you may have (or need), some may be out-of-pocket. You—and your adviser—need to factor all this in.

Do you believe I should evaluate my financial program based on the same criteria as we've used in the past? What about cash flow and not just ROI? Does your adviser think that longevity means you could have a slightly higher tolerance for risk?

What about issues like outliving my money and the need for income? Is your adviser aware of your goals, interests, or activities? Might some of them involve costs you should factor in?

Are you aware of SuperAging? Even if your adviser doesn't know about the exact phrase, how aware are they of longevity and its implications for financial planning? Some of the most exciting developments in extending the human lifespan will involve higher costs. How can your adviser help you make sure that you'll be in a position to afford the new drugs or high-tech solutions?

Have you taken any steps to improve or upgrade your knowledge and skills as they specifically relate to the topic of aging? Has your adviser taken any training programs or obtained a seniors designation or certification of any kind?

Do you think you need more expertise on your team to really help me? Is your adviser prepared to be the quarterback of a team that can bring more experience and expertise to the issue? Can they bring in a real estate specialist if required? An occupational therapist who can audit your home for its aging-in-place potential and map out a plan for renovation? A high-tech expert? A lifestyle reinvention coach? Or is it up to you to find these people?

The answers to these questions will give you a lot of insight into how well your planner is equipped—in terms of both abilities and attitudes—to meet your future needs as a SuperAger. You can also use these questions to evaluate any new financial advisers.

IS IT TIME TO SAY GOODBYE?

Good warning signs that it's time to say goodbye to your doctor or financial adviser:

- ❑ Poor listening skills
- ❑ Casual about service (hard to get hold of, vague about explaining fees)
- ❑ Dismissive or patronizing about your concerns and treats them as something you shouldn't trouble yourself with

Above all, your doctor and financial adviser should be supportive of your SuperAging program.

BUILD AWARENESS AROUND AGE-TECH AND HEALTHCARE

These two fields are exploding, with new products and services being released practically every day. For example:

Smart cooking appliances can adjust cooking times and temperatures based on the food being prepared. These devices often come with voice-activated controls, making them accessible for people who may have mobility problems or difficulty with manual settings.

AI-driven apps can help people plan meals tailored to their dietary needs and preferences. These apps can suggest recipes based on the ingredients available in the kitchen, automatically generate shopping lists, and offer online grocery-ordering options. For people managing specific health conditions, such as diabetes or hypertension, AI can recommend meals that align with their nutritional goals.

Wearable devices and remote monitoring systems are enabling remote healthcare delivery and telemedicine services. These technologies allow patients to monitor their health from the comfort of their homes while providing healthcare providers with real-time data on their conditions.

Capture your search terms or areas of interest here.

KEY TAKEAWAYS

Use this space to write down your key takeaways, notes to self, and anything else you'd like to remember from this chapter.

NEXT STEPS

Remember the honorary eighth pillar: *Accountability.* Fill in the blanks, giving yourself a reasonable time horizon. Be as specific as possible about the action and your reason(s) for undertaking it. Concrete whys help ensure follow-through.

In the next ________________, I will ____.

I'm going to do this because ____.

I'm also excited to ____.

FINDING A COMMUNITY THAT WORKS FOR YOU

According to the National Association of Realtors' 2024 *Home Buyers and Sellers Generational Trends Report*, one in five home buyers over the age of 60 are buying into age-restricted (usually 55+) communities.

CHAPTER 7

ATTACHMENT

WHY GETTING ATTACHED IS GOOD FOR YOU

Having a strong social network with meaningful relationships is no longer just an abstract "good thing" that you may or may not enjoy, but can't do much about. In the world of SuperAging, it's a vital component of "getting older without getting old," and it is very attainable!

Social isolation and loneliness are associated with a significant increase in the risk of premature death from all causes—a risk that's as great as smoking 15 cigarettes a day or being at an unhealthy weight. For those who are socially isolated, there's a 50% increase in the risk of having dementia and about a 30% increase in the risk of heart disease or stroke. There are significantly higher rates of depression, poor sleep quality, and cognitive decline.

None of these outcomes is particularly surprising, but why do social isolation and loneliness cause such damage? One explanation is behavioral and not connected to biological or clinical causes: People who are isolated are more likely to slip into health-jeopardizing behaviors (poor diet, inactivity) and remain trapped in them because they do not have anyone encouraging and motivating them toward healthier options.

Attachment, then, is not just a desirable environmental or behavioral condition, but a biological necessity to healthier aging and longevity.

MAKE ATTACHMENT PART OF YOUR SUPERAGING PROGRAM

In this section, you will learn how to:

- ☐ **Strengthen your attachments.**
- ☐ **Use digital technology.**
- ☐ **Grow your network.**

ASSESS YOUR ATTACHMENTS

Spend some time considering the main relationships in your life. Think about your spouse/partner, friends, children, even grandchildren or adult siblings. Which relationships need some care? Which relationships are you proudest of?

GAZE INTO EACH OTHER'S EYES

Looking for a way to strengthen a romantic attachment? Gaze into each other's eyes. Scientists have found that staring into another person's eyes for two minutes can heighten feelings of attraction and affection.

STRENGTHEN YOUR RELATIONSHIPS

The strategies below aren't revolutionary, but they are straightforward and definitely capable of enhancing the bond between you and your loved one or friend.

- ❑ **Spend time together.**
- ❑ **Listen actively.** Ask follow-up questions.
- ❑ **Be present.** Put down your phone.
- ❑ **Develop a shared interest.** Perhaps you both like crime shows, or maybe you meet for a walk every day (Attachment + Activity!).
- ❑ **Celebrate accomplishments.** Be a cheerleader.
- ❑ **Try new things.** Flip back to p. 105 and see whether any of the activities you listed would benefit from a buddy.
- ❑ **Say "please" and "thank you."** Over time, it becomes easy to take people for granted, and paradoxically we often have the shortest amount of patience for those we see most often.
- ❑ **Reminisce about past experiences.**
- ❑ **Be vulnerable.** Be willing to open up and share.

HOW WILL YOU BUILD STRONGER RELATIONSHIPS?

Pick two relationships you want to strengthen (maybe referring back to what you wrote on p. 133). List concrete actions you'll take to help cultivate your relationships with those people. Remember, too, that cultivating and strengthening relationships take time.

Relationship #1:

Strategies for strengthening your relationship:

Relationship #2:

Strategies for strengthening your relationship:

AUDIT YOUR WEAK TIES

In 1973, sociologist Mark Granovetter released a groundbreaking paper, in which he argued for the importance of "weak ties," particularly as they relate to careers and networking. Strong ties are the big relationships in our lives, like spouses or close friends. But what was surprising was the significance of weak ties. Basically, even casual acquaintances bestow positive benefits to our lives—indeed, a robust social network is composed of both strong and weak ties. The quality of your relationships matters, but so does the quantity.

Consider your casual acquaintances, or weak ties. You might include neighbors, baristas, fellow commuters, and people you see regularly at the gym or grocery store. Your goal here is to get a sense of the breadth and depth of your social network. Jot down the folks who come to mind—those you look forward to seeing.

LIFELONG FRIENDS

In Okinawa, people consciously and deliberately create a future support network. The *moai* is a support circle of about five friends, who form in childhood and pledge to be there for each other throughout their lives.

The concept originated hundreds of years ago as a mechanism for enabling a village's financial support system by pooling resources for large projects or public works. It gradually morphed into a system of small, intimate circles of friends offering mutual support. Members of the moai meet, often daily, to share meals, exchange ideas, gossip, and entertain. Over 40% of Okinawans are in one or more moai, and some moais have lasted more than 90 years.

USE DIGITAL TECHNOLOGY

Some studies have shown that older individuals who use the internet more have higher perceptions of self-efficacy and lower levels of cognitive decline. SuperAgers are tech-savvy and eager users of the internet for everything from social network sites to peer support chat groups to online gaming.

A 2016 study by the government of British Columbia identified eight different technologies that can alleviate social isolation:

- ❑ General information and communications (i.e., searching for information, interacting with content)
- ❑ Video games
- ❑ Robotics
- ❑ Social network sites
- ❑ Personal reminder information and social management systems
- ❑ Peer support chat rooms
- ❑ Telehealth
- ❑ 3D virtual environments

TEST OUT A NEW TECHNOLOGY

Pick a digital technology from the list on the previous page that you've never tried before, and give it a whirl. Then come back to this page to write about what you picked, how it went, and whether you felt more connected (no pun intended).

VOLUNTEER VIRTUALLY

When we think of volunteering, we usually think about going somewhere and physically lending a hand. But virtual volunteering enables you to do good without leaving your home. Search "virtual volunteering," or try VolunteerMatch.org, which lets you sort opportunities by different criteria, including cause, skills required, location, and in-person/virtual.

CONSIDER HOME SHARING

The concept of home sharing is growing rapidly in popularity, as a way to both reduce costs and combat isolation. Both are important pillars of the SuperAging strategy to "get older without getting old." They're represented by two of our seven *A*'s—Autonomy, which includes financial independence, and Attachment, which speaks to the role of social connection in promoting longevity. Benefits of home sharing include cost savings, increased social interaction, and enhanced safety. Would you share your home? If so, with whom? If not, what would it take to change your mind?

MAKE NEW FRIENDS AND GROW YOUR NETWORK

Let's look at some expert-backed tips for making new friends and building social networks as we age. What we love about these tips is the way they dovetail with the other pillars of SuperAging; the pillars really are interconnected.

- ❑ **Leverage hobbies and interests.** Community centers and local libraries often host activities and classes tailored to older adults, providing a relaxed environment to meet people with similar passions; you can also try online resources like Meetup.com.
- ❑ **Volunteer for a cause you care about.** Whether you choose to support a local food bank, animal shelter, or hospital, working alongside others creates opportunities to forge deeper connections through shared experiences and similar values.
- ❑ **Join fitness or wellness groups.** Exercise classes such as yoga, tai chi, or walking clubs offer more than just physical benefits—they're also great social opportunities. Regularly attending group fitness classes provides consistency, allowing you to get to know people over time.
- ❑ **Explore educational opportunities.** Enrolling in a class not only stimulates the mind but also puts you in a social environment with others who are eager to learn. This setting naturally encourages discussion and relationship-building.
- ❑ **Attend social events or meetups.** Bookstores, community centers, and places of worship often host activities such as literary events, game nights, potlucks, or movie screenings. These events create a low-pressure environment for people to meet and mingle.
- ❑ **Rekindle old friendships.** Reaching out to old friends, former colleagues, or acquaintances can be an easy way to reestablish meaningful relationships. Social media makes reconnecting with past connections easier than ever.
- ❑ **Participate in religious or spiritual groups.** Many of us find companionship and a sense of belonging in religious or spiritual groups. These communities often provide built-in support

systems, offering opportunities for fellowship, social gatherings, and volunteering.

- ❑ **Be open—and pack your patience.** Whether it's getting to know your neighbors better or turning professional relationships into more personal ones, building new relationships can take time, so try not to get discouraged if they don't deepen immediately. Instead, allow relationships to develop naturally and focus on enjoying the process of meeting, and getting to know, new people.

HOW WILL YOU GROW YOUR NETWORK?

Pick one of the strategies listed above to try to grow your network. Use the space below to make notes as part of your planning and to reflect once you've tried the strategy.

Strategy: ____________________

What do you plan to do? How? When? Where? Be specific to ensure follow-through.

____

____

____

____

____

Was your strategy successful? ____________________

____

____

____

Would you try this strategy again? Why or why not? ____________________

____

____

____

____

KEY TAKEAWAYS

Use this space to write down your key takeaways, notes to self, and anything else you'd like to remember from this chapter.

NEXT STEPS

Remember the honorary eighth pillar: *Accountability.* Fill in the blanks, giving yourself a reasonable time horizon. Be as specific as possible about the action and your reason(s) for undertaking it. Concrete whys help ensure follow-through.

In the next __________________________, I will ____.

I'm going to do this because ____.

I'm also excited to ____.

COMEDIAN AT AGE 90

According to the *Guinness Book of World Records*, D'yan Forest is the world's oldest working female comedian, a career she began at age 71. In addition to jokes about her childhood, cabaret career in Paris, and bisexuality, her show often includes parody songs on her ukulele, such as transforming "I'm Singing in the Rain" into "I'm Swinging on the Seine."

CHAPTER 8

AVOIDANCE

HOW TO AVOID THE BIG PROBLEMS

If you've reached the stage where SuperAging is what's next, you've already lived enough years to know that life is full of problems and often the best strategy is to roll with the punches. So this Avoidance list is limited only to big issues that can impede SuperAging if not dealt with:

1. Ageism in general, and in the workplace in particular.
2. Frauds and scams are not a brand-new topic, but with a whole new digital generation of sophistication, they are more alarming than ever.
3. Obsolete advisers are perhaps not obvious, but the phenomenon is real and could seriously slow you down. Use our checklists in the "Autonomy" chapter to ensure that your doctor and financial adviser in particular are serving you and your needs.

4. We should also try to tune out negative perceptions about aging itself. Remember the flip side of this: Positivity promotes better health and longevity.

It's worth noting that the problems on our Avoidance list, while potentially serious, are more than outweighed by the opportunities created by the SuperAging revolution. They can't really stand in its way. That's why we deliberately used the relatively mild word "avoidance" instead of some more drastic term. With enough knowledge and attention to the details, you can work around them! We'll show you how to get started.

MAKE AVOIDANCE PART OF YOUR SUPERAGING PROGRAM

In this section, you will learn how to:

- ❑ **Recognize ageism in the workplace, in media, and in politics.**
- ❑ **Confront ageist stereotypes.**
- ❑ **Avoid scams and stay safe online.**

BE ATTUNED TO AGEISM

Ageism is no longer just a mild sociocultural attitude. It has hardened and become more active and concrete, and therefore it threatens the SuperAging mission.

- **Ageism in the workplace.** Some progress has been made, driven particularly by an emerging shortage of workers and the increasingly desperate need for companies to retain older workers and even recruit them back out of retirement. But strong resistance remains, and it's a serious impediment to SuperAgers who want to work past 65. Write about a time you've seen ageism in the workplace.

- **Ageism in the marketplace.** On this front, it's more a matter of ignorance and indifference than malice. Marketers have massively underestimated the scale and power of SuperAgers as consumers, which in turn has retarded the development of new and better products and services. The tide is turning (slowly, slowly), but it's up to SuperAgers to create a real push here. When have you seen a product or marketing tactic that ignored or undervalued an older audience?

- **Ageism in the political arena.** This is where campaigns such as "OK, Boomer" are unambiguously harmful. There's always been a fight for the allocation of scarce government resources—childcare versus pensions, student-debt relief versus healthcare. But the campaign to portray Boomers as having hogged too many resources and deserving of little or nothing further can influence public policy against the rights and interests of SuperAgers, who are emphatically not at the end of the road. Think about a time when you've felt boxed out of the current political conversation. How did it feel?

These issues matter and require a response. You can undertake individual actions on the six other *A*'s, but you also need to be doing it in an environment that supports and encourages the SuperAging revolution. Ageism is a cancer to that environment. In fact, we could probably upgrade the *A* from Avoidance to Abolition in the case of ageism. It's that serious.

AGEISM IS EVERYWHERE

An AARP study found that 61% of workers aged 45 and older had experienced or witnessed some form of age-related discrimination. Of that group, more than 90% said that they "believe that such discrimination is common."

OCTOGENARIAN MODELS

Wang Deshun earned the nickname "world's hottest grandpa" after walking in a Beijing fashion show at age 80. Fun fact: He didn't start working out until he was almost 50. Fellow octogenarian Martha Stewart made waves when she appeared on the cover of the 2023 *Sports Illustrated* swimsuit issue at age 81, becoming the magazine's oldest cover star to date.

When you hear about accomplishments like these in our youth-oriented, looks-obsessed culture, what's your first reaction? Yay? No way? Somewhere in between? Be honest, but be mindful of how insidious ageism can be.

MAKE A LIST OF AGEIST STEREOTYPES

From being called "dear" or "young lady" to having people assume you don't know how to work an iPhone, ageist stereotypes abound. Use this space to write down ageist stereotypes you've encountered.

STOP STEREOTYPING YOURSELF

Avoid making self-deprecating comments about your age. Instead of being funny, jokes about "senior moments" center and draw attention to your age, implying that a person's age should be equated with a set of characteristics, or that getting older is negative. In addition, negative stereotypes about aging have been found to contribute to adverse health outcomes, including higher blood pressure and lower scores on cognitive tests.

COMBAT THE "TOO OLD" MENTALITY

The next time you hear someone say that a person is "too old" to be doing something, swap in another identity and see how it sounds. Would you ever say that someone is "too gay" or "too Latina"?

ASK THE MAGIC QUESTION

When dealing with healthcare professionals, financial advisers, and other service providers, ask the following question: *Are you aware of SuperAging?* Then notice the person's reaction. Do they seem genuinely curious and intrigued? Do they scoff, laugh, or otherwise respond dismissively? Do they nod knowingly and share their own insights? This simple question can help you gauge ageism and avoid obsolete advisers.

Find an opportunity to ask this question, then write about the reaction and response you got.

LOOK FOR AGEISM IN THE MEDIA

Advertising is working hard (if not intentionally or maliciously) to perpetuate DefaultAging as the defining condition of aging. In the ad world, getting older without getting old is a contradiction; getting older *means* getting old.

A lack of representation in the media hurts SuperAgers in two specific ways:

1. It hides the SuperAging revolution, which in turn spills over into more ageism in the workplace and the political arena (which we'll explore next).
2. It slows down the pace of developing new products and services, or inadequately communicates valuable ones, leading to less uptake.

Find an ad that's ageist, that portrays older consumers as weak, confused, staid, and cheap, for example. What was the ad for? How did it come across as ageist? If you can't find an ad that's ageist, discuss a brand's missed opportunity to market to SuperAgers.

CONSIDER YOUR RESPONSE

If you see an ad or commercial that displays ageism, consider the following menu of responses: File a formal complaint with regulators, file a complaint with the media where you saw the ad or commercial, or stop purchasing the product. You have more power than you think to end ageism!

AVOID FRAUD AND SCAMS

There are three simple strategies here:

- ❑ **Know what techniques are out there.** Periodically check with organizations like the AARP or CARP, which regularly report on the latest frauds and scams, and which in turn can link you to appropriate local resources, including law enforcement agencies that keep up to date and often issue advisories.
- ❑ **Know where to report a fraud, scam, or security breach if you think it's happened to you.** Alert your local police, who will know how to handle your complaint or to which other enforcement agency to route it. Since many frauds and scams may involve bank accounts or credit cards, any known (or even suspicious) activity should be reported immediately to the banks or credit card companies.
- ❑ **Build a defensive wall in the digital space.** Take action to protect yourself and to stay cybersafe.

STAY CYBERSAFE

Unfortunately, online fraud and scams continue to proliferate. Fighting them is, unfortunately, grunt work—an ongoing grind rather than a single overarching strategy. It means paying attention to a lot of nasty little things. But increasingly, there are many tech solutions that can help. Frauds and scams can be avoided, but the necessary homework can't.

Write about a fraud or scam that you've heard about, or that has happened to someone you know. How did the scam work? What was the fallout?

Here's some guidance on protecting yourself online:

- ❑ **Use strong, unique passwords.** Create strong passwords for each of your online accounts, using a mix of letters, numbers, and special characters. Consider using a password manager to generate and store complex passwords securely (see below for more info).
- ❑ **Enable two-factor authentication (2FA).** Adding an extra layer of security, such as a text-message code or an authentication app, can significantly reduce the risk of unauthorized access to your accounts.
- ❑ **Be cautious with emails, texts, and links.** Avoid clicking on links or downloading attachments from unknown sources. Verify the sender's identity and be wary of emails that create a sense of urgency or ask for personal information or make monetary requests.
- ❑ **Regularly update software.** Ensure that your operating system, browsers, and applications are up to date to protect against vulnerabilities that cybercriminals can exploit.
- ❑ **Let unfamiliar calls go to voicemail.** Don't answer any inbound phone call that shows just a phone number and no caller ID. There may be a very few exceptions, but the general rule of thumb should be if you can't see who's calling, don't take the call. Even better, program your smartphone to block that number in the future.
- ❑ **Monitor financial accounts.** Regularly check your bank statements, credit card bills, and other financial accounts for any suspicious activity. Report any discrepancies immediately.
- ❑ **Review privacy settings.** Regularly review and adjust the privacy settings on your social media accounts and other online services. Limit the amount of personal information you share publicly and be cautious about who can see your posts and personal details. Many platforms offer settings that allow you to control who can view your profile, posts, and contact information.
- ❑ **Consider an identity-theft-protection program.** There are many services that can patrol the internet, including the dark web, to see if your Social Security number, bank accounts, or credit cards have been compromised.

PROTECT YOUR PASSWORDS

According to *Wired*, the most common passwords are "password" and "123456." But even if you have strong passwords for every site you visit (which you should!), it's impossible to remember them all. Enter a passport manager, which allows you to save and store unique passwords. Many browsers now offer this feature, or you can sign up for a service like 1Password.

SAFEGUARD YOUR INFORMATION

List your cybersafe to-dos, including programs to research or sources to consult.

THINK TWICE ABOUT SCANNING THAT QR CODE

In 2023, the US Federal Trade Commission issued a warning about QR codes, noting that scammers can put fake codes atop or inside real ones. As always, think before you click. The FTC also recommends that people carefully examine URLs and follow up by phone or website, especially in the event they receive an urgent message from a company asking them to take immediate action.

EDUCATE YOURSELF

According to data released by the FBI, North Americans between the ages of 30 and 49 are more likely to fall victim to investment scammers than those who are older. If anything, such a statistic should make us even more vigilant, since the fact that younger generations are just as susceptible shows how skilled the scammers are.

The rapidity with which new scams occur is astonishing. As part of your Awareness activities, dedicate some amount of time each month to researching new scams and learning how to protect yourself. List your trusted sources for such information here.

KEY TAKEAWAYS

Use this space to write down your key takeaways, notes to self, and anything else you'd like to remember from this chapter.

NEXT STEPS

Remember the honorary eighth pillar: *Accountability.* Fill in the blanks, giving yourself a reasonable time horizon. Be as specific as possible about the action and your reason(s) for undertaking it. Concrete whys help ensure follow-through.

In the next ____________, I will ____

____

____.

I'm going to do this because ____

____

____.

I'm also excited to ____

____

____.

EXPLORER AT 75

Barbara Hillary was the first Black woman to visit the North Pole when she arrived in April 2007 at age 75. To achieve this goal, she overcame significant challenges, including cancer-related health issues. A few years later, she became the first Black woman to visit the South Pole, at age 79. Inspired by what she saw on her travels, she became a motivational speaker and climate-change activist.

CHAPTER 9

YOU'RE A SUPERAGER NOW!

Congratulations! Having completed this workbook, you've gotten a thorough grounding in the seven pillars—and you now have the tools you need to continue being a part of the SuperAging revolution. You'll be able to get older without getting old!

Based on your answers to the activities, you may wish to set up a formal action plan and system of to-do lists. You may wish to go deeper into a pillar or topic than we did here. No matter what, you have a new perspective. (To check that new perspective, here's your reminder to redo the quizzes you took in chapter 2 on Attitude.)

It is possible to live much longer. And it is possible to experience those extra years as a time of growth, development, and accomplishment as opposed to decline and retreat. What's more, that growth and development is made even more exciting precisely because of the lifetime of learning and experience you've already gained. That's why we make no apology for the "age" part of SuperAging. It's not something to hide or work around; it's an essential component to making the future so rich. Your accumulated knowledge and wisdom (including the mistakes you've learned from) are priceless building blocks for a future that has plenty of capacity to be even more fulfilling.

You're part of a worldwide community now, a community that is carrying out the most profound and far-reaching social development in history: the redefinition of aging itself.

Thank you for embracing SuperAging. It's going to be an exciting future for all of us!

WHAT'S CHANGED FOR YOU?

What's been your biggest change or revelation since starting this workbook? Stronger relationships? New exercise routine? Brighter outlook?

KEEP LEARNING ABOUT SUPERAGING

If you haven't done so, please take a look at our book, *SuperAging: Getting Older Without Getting Old*, which goes deep into the science and research behind the seven pillars in this workbook. As we've mentioned throughout, our companion website, SuperAgingNews.com, is an essential component as well. SuperAging is a topic around which something new is happening all the time—new research and discoveries, new products and services, new ways to meet like-minded people—and the internet is obviously the best way to stay updated. SuperAging News will offer more detailed resources for the topics we've covered here, as well as news, podcasts, videos (also see our YouTube channel!), interviews with experts, and an entire interactive community where you, as a SuperAger, can share information and ideas with other SuperAgers. On the SuperAging News website, SuperAgingNews.com, you'll also find links to our social media accounts like Facebook and Instagram. We have a dynamic and growing community on Facebook.

FINAL TAKEAWAYS

Use this space to write down your key takeaways, notes to self, and anything else you'd like to remember from this workbook.

WHAT'S NEXT?

Use this space to write down your next steps, from revisiting some of the content you might have bookmarked to finding a new physician to gaining a professional certification. We wish you joy and luck on your SuperAging journey!

REFERENCES

INTRODUCTION

SuperAging News. "Never Say Never: 12 SuperAgers Who Continued to Make Their Mark Later in Life." Accessed April 10, 2025. https://superagingnews.com/never-say-never-12-superagers-who-continued-to-make-their-mark-later-in-life/.

CHAPTER 1: THE 7 A'S OF SUPERAGING

Blumberg, Yoni. "Millennials Spend Less Than Previous Generations Because They Literally Have Less Money, Fed Says." CNBC, December 4, 2018. https://www.cnbc.com/2018/12/04/millennials-spend-less-because-theyre-poorer-federal-reserve-says.html.

Clark, Amie. "Life on a College or University Campus—an Alternative Retirement Destination." Senior List, April 1, 2022. https://www.theseniorlist.com/retirement/best/university/.

Estella's Brilliant Bus. Accessed April 10, 2025. https://estellasbrilliantbus.org/index.html.

Pawlowski, A. "Optimists Live Longer, Study Finds. Here's How to Boost Positive Thinking." *Today*, August 26, 2019. https://www.today.com/health/how-live-longer-study-links-optimism-longevity-t161337.

CHAPTER 2: ATTITUDE

Alimujiang, Aliya, Ashley Wiensch, Jonathan Boss, et al. "Association Between Life Purpose and Mortality Among US Adults Older Than 50 Years." JAMA Network (May 24, 2019). https://jamanetwork.com/journals/jamanetworkopen/fullarticle/2734064.

BU School of Medicine. "New Evidence That Optimists Live Longer." August 26, 2019. https://www.bumc.bu.edu/busm/2019/08/26/new-evidence-that-optimists-live-longer/.

Christensen, Kaare, Anne Maria Herskind, and James W. Vaupel. "Why Danes Are Smug: Comparative Study of Life Satisfaction in the European Union." *BMJ* 333, no. 7582 (2006): 1289–91. https://www.ncbi.nlm.nih.gov/pmc/articles/PMC1761170/.

Cravit, David. "J. P. Morgan Tells Its Advisors to Assume Retirees Will Live to 100." *Everything Zoomer*, April 18, 2022. https://www.everythingzoomer.com/health/longevity-wellness/2022/04/18/j-p-morgan-tells-its-advisors-to-assume-retirees-will-live-to-100.

Fielding, Sarah. "Why 1 in 5 Adults Over Age 50 Say Their Sex Life Is Way More Exciting Now." *mbgRelationships*, June 23, 2019. https://www.mindbodygreen.com/articles/how-often-people-have-sex-after-50-60-70-and-older-and-how-to-increase-frequency/.

Fogelman, Nia, and Turhan Canli. "'Purpose in Life' as a Psychosocial Resource in Healthy Aging: An Examination of Cortisol Baseline Levels and Response to the Trier Social Stress Test." *npj Aging*, September 28, 2015. https://www.nature.com/articles/npjamd20156.

Gander, Kashmira. "Religious People Live Four Years Longer on Average: Study." *Newsweek*, June 14, 2018. https://www.newsweek.com/religious-people-live-four-years-longer-average-study-shows-976050.

Hall, Nicholas. "Is Feeling Better as Easy as ABC?" *Positive Psychology News*, June 6, 2007. https://positivepsychologynews.com/news/nicholas-hall/20070606273.

Hayes, Kim. "How Is Your Emodiversity?" *AARP*, June 27, 2017. https://www.aarp.org/health/conditions-treatments/info-2017/positive-emotions-may-reduce-inflammation-fd.html.

Hennefield, Laura, Laura M. Talpey, and Lori Markson. "When Positive Outcomes and Reality Collide: Children Prefer Optimists as Social Partners." *Cognitive Development* 59 (2021). https://www.ncbi.nlm.nih.gov/pmc/articles/PMC8478345/.

Independent. "LL Cool J: 'I was hanging out with some of the most dangerous characters in New York'." Accessed April 10, 2025. https://www.the-independent.com/arts-entertainment/music/features/ll-cool-j-interview-ncis-the-force-album-b2608135.html.

Klein, Jessica. "Are Baby Boomers Having the Best Time in Bed?" *BBC News*, April 21, 2022. https://www.bbc.com/worklife/article/20220420-are-baby-boomers-having-the-best-time-in-bed.

Mathur, Maya B., Elissa Epel, Shelley Kind, Manisha Desai, Christine G. Parks, Dale P. Sandler, and Nayer Khazeni. "Perceived Stress and Telomere Length: A Systematic Review, Meta-analysis, and Methodologic Considerations for Advancing the Field." *Brain, Behavior, and Immunity* 54 (May 2016): 158–69. https://www.sciencedirect.com/science/article/pii/S088915911630023X?via%3Dihub.

National Library of Medicine. "Well-being and Anticipation for Future Positive Events: Evidences from an fMRI Study." Accessed April 10, 2025. https://pmc.ncbi.nlm.nih.gov/articles/PMC5767250/.

Plomin, Richard, Michael F. Scheier, C. S. Bergeman, N. L. Pedersen, J. R. Nesselroade, and G. E. McClearn. "Optimism, Pessimism, and Mental Health: A Twin/Adoption Analysis." *Personality and Individual Differences* 13, no. 8 (August 1992): 921–30. https://www.sciencedirect.com/science/article/abs/pii/019188699290009E.

Robson, David. "Can You Think Yourself Young?" *Guardian*, January 2, 2022. https://www.theguardian.com/science/2022/jan/02/can-you-think-yourself-young-ageing-psychology.

Rosenthal, Jack. "Language: What Will You Call Me When I'm 64?" *New York Times*, July 27, 2007. https://www.nytimes.com/2007/07/22/opinion/22iht-edrosenthal.1.6767016.html.

Skipper, Clay. "Why Your Brain Is Wired for Pessimism—and What You Can Do to Fix It." *GQ*, September 23, 2018. https://www.gq.com/story/how-to-be-more-optimistic.

SuperAging News. "9 Expert Tips to Protect Your Mental Health . . . and Your Lifespan." Accessed April 10, 2025. https://superagingnews.com/self-care-9-expert-tips-to-protect-your-mental-health-and-your-lifespan/

SuperAging News. "Is There Such a Thing as Learning How to Be an Optimist?" Accessed April 10, 2025. https://superagingnews.com/is-there-such-a-thing-as-learning-how-to-be-an-optimist/.

SuperAging News. "World Happiness Report Finds Massive Difference Between Older and Younger People." Accessed April 10, 2025. https://superagingnews.com/world-happiness-report-finds-massive-difference-between-older-younger-people/.

Tessler Lindau, Stacy, et al. "A Study of Sexuality and Health Among Older Adults in the United States." *New England Journal of Medicine*, August 23, 2007. https://www.nejm.org/doi/full/10.1056/nejmoa067423.

"Thinking Positively About Aging Extends Life More Than Exercise and Not Smoking." *YaleNews*, July 29, 2002. https://news.yale.edu/2002/07/29/thinking-positively-about-aging-extends-life-more-exercise-and-not-smoking.

University of Kansas. "People by Nature Are Universally Optimistic, Study Shows." *ScienceDaily*, May 25, 2009. https://www.sciencedaily.com/releases/2009/05/090524122539.htm.

CHAPTER 3: AWARENESS

Daily Mail. "101-year-old college student prepares to graduate alongside her granddaughter 82 years after she dropped out when she fell pregnant with the first of her 12 children." Accessed April 10, 2025. https://www.dailymail.co.uk/news/article-12895591/Centenarian-Sarah-Simpkins-college-student-granddaughter.html.

SuperAging News. "Can Taking a Vacation Help You Live Longer?" Accessed April 10, 2025. https://superagingnews.com/can-taking-a-vacation-help-you-live-longer-heres-what-the-experts-say/.

SuperAging News. "Debunking 8 Medical Myths About Dementia and Alzheimer's Disease." Accessed April 10, 2025. https://superagingnews.com/debunking-8-medical-myths-about-dementia-and-alzheimers-disease/.

SuperAging News. "Experts Say You Should Exercise in Short Bursts and Before Bed." Accessed April 10, 2025. https://superagingnews.com/experts-say-you-should-exercise-in-short-bursts-and-before-bed/.

CHAPTER 4: ACTIVITY

Baker, Joseph, et al. "Sport Participation and Positive Development in Older Persons." *European Review of Aging and Physical Activity* 7 (2010). https://eurapa.biomedcentral.com/articles/10.1007/s11556-009-0054-9.

Browse by Collection. DIYbiosphere, 2022. https://sphere.diybio.org/.

Bryant, Erin. "Lack of Sleep in Middle Age May Increase Dementia Risk." National Institutes of Health, April 27, 2021. https://www.nih.gov/news-events/nih-research-matters/lack-sleep-middle-age-may-increase-dementia-risk.

Elhuyar Foundation. "Study on 90-Year-Olds Reveals the Benefits of Strength Training." *ScienceDaily*, September 27, 2013. https://www.sciencedaily.com/releases/2013/09/130927092350.htm#.

"From Grinders to Biohackers: Where Medical Technology Meets Body Modification." *Medical Technology*, January 2022. https://medical-technology.nridigital.com/medical_technology_jan20/from_grinders_to_biohackers_where_medical_technology_meets_body_modification.

The Harvard Gazette. "Berries keep your brain sharp." Accessed April 10, 2025. https://news.harvard.edu/gazette/story/2012/04/berries-keep-your-brain-sharp/.

Harvard Health Publishing. "Fruit of the Month: Berries." Accessed April 10, 2025. https://www.health.harvard.edu/heart-health/fruit-of-the-month-berries.

Healthline. "11 Evidence-Based Health Benefits of Eating Fish." Accessed April 10, 2025. https://www.healthline.com/nutrition/11-health-benefits-of-fish%23TOC_TITLE_HDR_3.

Healthline Editorial Team. "Why It's Never Too Late to Start Exercising." *Healthline*, September 4, 2019.

https://www.healthline.com/health-news/why-its-never-too-late-to-start-exercising.

Herskind, Anne Maria, Matt Mcgue, Niels Vilstrup Holm, and Thorkild I. A. Sørenson. "The Heritability of Human Longevity: A Population-Based Study of 2,872 Danish Twin Pairs Born 1870–1900." *Human Genetics* 97, no. 3 (April 1996): 319–23. https://www.researchgate.net/publication/14416947_The_heritability_of_human_longevity_A_population-based_study_of_2872_Danish_twin_pairs_born_1870-1900.

Huang, Jiaqi, et al. "Association Between Plant and Animal Protein Intake and Overall and Cause-Specific Mortality." *JAMA Internal Medicine* 180, no. 9 (2020): 1173–84. https://pubmed.ncbi.nlm.nih.gov/32658243/.

Klatsky, Arthur L. "Moderate Drinking and Reduced Risk of Heart Disease." *Alcohol Research & Health* 23, no. 1 (1999): 15–24. https://www.ncbi.nlm.nih.gov/pmc/articles/PMC6761693/.

LaCroix, Andrea Z. et al. "Does Walking Decrease the Risk of Cardiovascular Disease Hospitalizations and Death in Older Adults?" *Journal of the American Geriatrics Society* 44, no. 2 (February 1996): 113–20. https://agsjournals.onlinelibrary.wiley.com/doi/abs/10.1111/j.1532-5415.1996.tb02425.x.

Lanza, Ian R. et al. "Chronic Caloric Restriction Preserves Mitochondrial Function in Senescence Without Increasing Mitochondrial Biogenesis." *Cell Metabolism* 16, no. 6 (2012): 777–78. https://www.ncbi.nlm.nih.gov/pmc/articles/PMC3544078/.

Lineaweaver, Nicky. "Patients Are Transforming from Passive Recipients of Healthcare Services to Active Participants in Their Own Health." *Yahoo! News*, July 11, 2019. https://news.yahoo.com/patients-transforming-passive-recipients-healthcare-050000224.html.

Maki, Jessica. "Berries Delay Memory Decline in Adults." *SciTechDaily*, April 27, 2012. https://scitechdaily.com/berries-delay-memory-decline-in-adults/.

Mazzotti, Diego Robles, et al. "Human Longevity Is Associated with Regular Sleep Patterns, Maintenance of Slow Wave Sleep and Favorable Lipid Profile." *Frontiers in Aging Neuroscience* 6, no. 134 (2014). https://www.ncbi.nlm.nih.gov/pmc/articles/PMC4067693/.

McKeehan, Nick. "Loneliness and the Risk of Dementia." *Cognitive Vitality* (blog), April 16, 2019. https://www.alzdiscovery.org/cognitive-vitality/blog/loneliness-and-the-risk-of-dementia.

Millard, Elizabeth. "You May Need Less Daily Activity to Help You Live Longer Than You Think." *Verywell Fit*, December 18, 2020. https://www.verywellfit.com/you-may-need-less-daily-activity-than-you-think-5092758.

Murez, Cara. "This Balance Test May Predict Longevity." *HealthDay*, June 22, 2022. https://www.medicinenet.com/script/main/art.asp?articlekey=278013.

National Library of Medicine. "Randomized Controlled Trial of Social Ballroom Dancing and Treadmill Walking: Preliminary Findings on Executive Function and Neuroplasticity From Dementia-at-Risk Older Adults." Accessed April 10, 2025. https://pmc.ncbi.nlm.nih.gov/articles/PMC10264554/.

New York Times. "Older Adults Do Not Benefit From Moderate Drinking, Large Study Finds." Accessed April 10, 2025. https://www.nytimes.com/2024/08/12/health/alcohol-cancer-heart-disease.html.

"Nutrigenomics: The Basics." Nutrition Society, November 19, 2018. https://www.nutritionsociety.org/blog/nutrigenomics-basics.

Physicians Committee for Responsible Medicine. "Consuming More Protein from Plants Associated with Longer Life." *Health and Nutrition News*, July 23, 2020. https://www.pcrm.org/news/health-nutrition/consuming-more-protein-plants-associated-longer-life.

ResearchGate. "Psychological benefits of hobby engagement in older age: a longitudinal cross-country analysis of 93,263 older adults in 16 countries." Accessed April 10, 2025. https://www.researchgate.net/publication/366160647_Psychological_benefits_of_hobby_engagement_in_older_age_a_longitudinal_cross-country_analysis_of_93263_older_adults_in_16_countries.

Reynolds, Gretchen. "Brisk Walking Is Good for the Aging Brain." *New York Times*, March 31, 2021. https://www.nytimes.com/2021/03/31/well/move/seniors-memory-walking.html.

Reynolds, Gretchen. "Walking Just 10 Minutes a Day May Lead to a Longer Life." *New York Times*, January 26, 2022. https://www.nytimes.com/2022/01/26/well/10-minutes-walking-exercise.html#.

Robertson, Sally. "Walking for Just 20 Minutes a Day May Reduce Death Risk." *News Medical Life Sciences*, January 15, 2015. https://www.news-medical.net/news/20150115/Walking-for-just-20-minutes-a-day-may-reduce-death-risk.aspx.

Stenner, Brad J., Jonathan D. Buckley, and Amber D. Mosewich. "Reasons Why Older Adults Play Sport: A Systemic Review." *Journal of Sport and Health Science* 9, no. 6 (2020): 530–41. https://pubmed.ncbi.nlm.nih.gov/33308804/.

"Study Finds Association Between Sleep Problems and Dementia." National Heart, Lung, and Blood Institute, July 2, 2021. https://www.nhlbi.nih.gov/news/2021/study-finds-association-between-sleep-problems-and-dementia#.

SuperAging News. "Can You Stand On One Leg for 10 Seconds?" Accessed April 10, 2025. https://superagingnews.com/can-you-stand-on-one-leg-for-10-seconds/.

SuperAging News. "Easy Ways to Add More Longevity Foods into Your Diet." Accessed April 10, 2025. https://superagingnews.com/healthy-hacks-easy-ways-to-add-more-longevity-foods-into-your-diet/.

SuperAging News. "Food as Medicine: Healthy Herbs and Super Spices." Accessed April 10, 2025. https://superagingnews.com/food-as-medicine-healthy-herbs-and-super-spices/.

SuperAging News. "Foods to Help You Live Longer, Stronger, Better." Accessed April 10, 2025. https://superagingnews.com/foods-to-help-you-live-longer-stronger-better/.

SuperAging News. "The Role of Protein Quality in Combatting Muscle Loss." Accessed April 10, 2025. https://superagingnews.com/healthy-aging-the-role-of-protein-quality-in-combatting-muscle-loss/.

SuperAging News. "Want to Live Longer? Read More Books." Accessed April 10, 2025. https://superagingnews.com/want-to-live-longer-read-more-books/.

Van Gelder, B. M. et al. "Coffee Consumption Is Inversely Associated with Cognitive Decline in Elderly European Men: The FINE Study." *European Journal of Clinical Nutrition* 61, no. 2 (2007): 226–32. https://pubmed.ncbi.nlm.nih.gov/16929246/.

Vogue. "Restarting My Childhood Hobby Changed My Life." Accessed April 10, 2025. https://www.vogue.com/article/restarting-my-childhood-hobby-changed-my-life-it-can-help-you-too.

Zylberberg, Shawn. "Aiming to Live Past 90? Moderate Wine Consumption Could Help." *Wine Spectator*, March 4, 2020. https://www.winespectator.com/articles/aiming-to-live-past-90-moderate-wine-consumption-could-help#.

CHAPTER 5: ACCOMPLISHMENT

CNN. "Yasmeen Lari, 'starchitect' turned social engineer, wins one of architecture's most coveted prizes." Accessed April 10, 2025. https://www.cnn.com/style/article/yasmeen-lari-riba-royal-gold-medal/index.html.

NPR. "He always wanted a Ph.D. in physics. He finally earned it at 89." Accessed April 10, 2025. https://www.npr.org/2021/11/07/1052005447/brown-university-89-phd-physics-dream.

SuperAging News. "Guess What's the Fastest Growing Segment of the Workforce?" Accessed April 10, 2025. https://superagingnews.com/guess-whats-the-fastest-growing-segment-of-the-workforce-hint-not-gen-z/.

SuperAging News. "Meet 10 Entrepreneurs Over 60." Accessed April 10, 2025. https://superagingnews.com/meet-10-entrepreneurs-over-60-the-trend-is-just-getting-started/.

SuperAging News. "More Americans Want to Start a Business Than Retire." Accessed April 10, 2025. https://superagingnews.com/more-americans-want-to-start-a-business-than-retire/.

CHAPTER 6: AUTONOMY

Mount Sinai. "How and when to get rid of unused medicines." Accessed April 10, 2025. https://www.mountsinai.org/health-library/selfcare-instructions/how-and-when-to-get-rid-of-unused-medicines.

New York Times. "At 90, William Shatner becomes the oldest person to reach 'the final frontier.'" Accessed April 10, 2025. https://www.nytimes.com/2021/10/13/science/william-shatner-space.html.

SuperAging News. "6 Ways Artificial Intelligence Is Paving the Way to Longer, Healthier Lives." Accessed April 10, 2025. https://superagingnews.com/6-ways-artificial-intelligence-is-paving-the-way-to-longer-healthier-lives/.

SuperAging News. "Age-Restricted Housing Developments Are Booming." Accessed April 10, 2025. https://superagingnews.com/age-restricted-housing-developments-are-booming/.

SuperAging News. "AI in the Kitchen." Accessed April 10, 2025. https://superagingnews.com/ai-in-the-kitchen-another-way-tech-could-help-with-aging-in-place/.

SuperAging News. "Do You Need a Longevity Team?" Accessed April 10, 2025. https://superagingnews.com/do-you-need-a-longevity-team-who-would-be-on-it/.

SuperAging News. "Investing for Longevity." Accessed April 10, 2025. https://superagingnews.com/investing-for-longevity-4-questions-to-ask-your-financial-adviser/.

CHAPTER 7: ATTACHMENT

Blue Zones. "Moai—This Tradition is Why Okinawan People Live Longer, Better." Accessed April 10, 2025. https://www.bluezones.com/2018/08/moai-this-tradition-is-why-okinawan-people-live-longer-better/.

New York Times. "7 Simple Exercises To Strengthen Your Relationship." Accessed April 10, 2025. https://www.nytimes.com/interactive/2022/02/11/well/strengthen-relationships.html.

New York Times. "How a 90-Year-Old Comedian Spends Her Sundays." Accessed April 10, 2025. https://www.nytimes.com/2024/09/14/nyregion/dyan-forest-comedian.html.

Stanford Report. "50 years on, Mark Granovetter's 'The Strength of Weak Ties' is stronger than ever." Accessed April 10, 2025. https://news.stanford.edu/stories/2023/07/strength-weak-ties.

SuperAging News. "Connections." Accessed April 10, 2025. https://superagingnews.com/connections-forging-meaningful-relationships-later-in-life/.

SuperAging News. "Golden Girls Come to Life." Accessed April 10, 2025. https://superagingnews.com/golden-girls-comes-to-life-home-sharing-a-growing-trend/.

SuperAging News. "How Tech Is Tackling Social Isolation." Accessed April 10, 2025. https://superagingnews.com/how-tech-is-tackling-social-isolation-check-out-these-new-solutions/.

SuperAging News. "Want to Live to 100?" Accessed April 10, 2025. https://superagingnews.com/want-to-live-to-100-heres-the-one-thing-you-should-never-do/.

University of Chicago. "Loneliness Triggers Cellular Changes That Can Cause Illness, Study Shows." *ScienceDaily*, November 23, 2015. https://www.sciencedaily.com/releases/2015/11/151123201925.htm.

CHAPTER 8: AVOIDANCE

AARP. "Age Discrimination Common in Workplace, Survey Says." Accessed April 10, 2025. https://www.aarp.org/work/age-discrimination/common-at-work/.

Federal Trade Commission. "Scammers hide harmful links in QR codes to steal your information." Accessed April 10, 2025. https://consumer.ftc.gov/consumer-alerts/2023/12/scammers-hide-harmful-links-qr-codes-steal-your-information.

Levy, Becca R. et al. "Ageism Amplifies Cost and Prevalence of Health Conditions." *Gerontologist* 60, no. 1 (February 2020): 174–81. https://academic.oup.com/gerontologist/article/60/1/174/5166947.

Martin, Ashley, and Michael S. North. "Equality for (Almost) All: Egalitarian Advocacy Predicts Lower Endorsement of Sexism and Racism, but Not Ageism." *Journal of Personality and Social Psychology* 123, no. 2 (January 2021). https://www.researchgate.net/publication/348609257_Equality_for_almost_all_Egalitarian_advocacy_predicts_lower_endorsement_of_sexism_and_racism_but_not_ageism.

National Cyber Security Centre. "Top tips for staying secure online." Accessed April 10, 2025. https://www.ncsc.gov.uk/collection/top-tips-for-staying-secure-online/password-managers.

New York Times. "An 80-Year-Old Model Reshapes China's Views on Aging." Accessed April 10, 2025. https://www.nytimes.com/2016/11/04/world/asia/china-wang-deshun-model-80.html.

Oxford Academic. "Reducing Cardiovascular Stress With Positive Self-Stereotypes of Aging." Accessed April 10, 2025. https://academic.oup.com/psychsocgerontology/article-abstract/55/4/P205/572850?redirectedFrom=fulltext&login=false.

Smithsonian Magazine. "Barbara Hillary, a Pioneering African-American Adventurer, Dies at 88." Accessed April 10, 2025. https://www.smithsonianmag.com/smart-news/barbara-hillary-pioneering-african-american-adventurer-has-died-180973663/.

SuperAging News. "Staying Cyber Safe." Accessed April 10, 2025. https://superagingnews.com/staying-cyber-safe-11-top-scams-and-how-not-to-fall-for-them/.

SuperAging News. "Surprise: Older People Are Not the Most Likely to Fall for Investment Scams." Accessed April 10, 2025. https://superagingnews.com/surprise-older-people-are-not-the-most-likely-to-fall-for-investment-scams/.

ABOUT THE AUTHORS

DAVID CRAVIT has an established profile and track record in reporting on aging and related issues. He is the author of three previous books: *The New Old,* which discusses how the Baby Boomers reinvented aging, *Beyond Age Rage,* which examines the so-called war of the generations, and (with Larry Wolf) *SuperAging: Getting Older Without Getting Old.* He is also cofounder of SuperAgingNews.com, which tracks the SuperAging revolution. He appears frequently on radio and television as a respected thought leader on the new trends and developments driving the emergence of SuperAging.

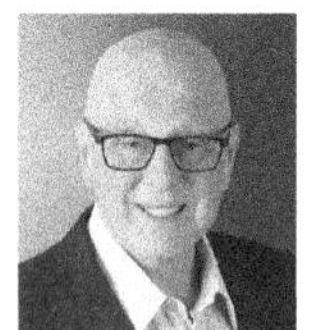

LARRY WOLF is the cofounder with David Cravit of SuperAgingNews.com, a rapidly growing digital information service delivering the latest news, ideas, and trends about living longer, healthier, and more fulfilling lives well into our 80s and 90s—and beyond. Larry's expertise is in identifying important consumer trends and capitalizing on them. As CEO of the Wolf Group, he has advised many Fortune 500 companies and governments on their branding and communications strategies. Larry saw the opportunity to change the way people approached aging itself, helping them become successful SuperAgers using the strategies and techniques that have guided his and David's lives.

www.ingramcontent.com/pod-product-compliance
Lightning Source LLC
Jackson TN
JSHW061329280725
88057JS00001B/1

* 9 7 8 1 9 6 4 7 2 1 2 1 7 *